Relating to Clients

The Therapeutic Relationship for Complementary Therapists

Su Fox

Jessica Kingsley Publishers
London and Philadelphia

First published in 2008
by Jessica Kingsley Publishers
116 Pentonville Road
London N1 9JB, UK
and
400 Market Street, Suite 400
Philadelphia, PA 19106, USA

www.jkp.com

Library of Congress Cataloging in Publication Data

Fox, Su, 1949-
Relating to clients : the therapeutic relationship for complementary therapists / Su Fox.
p. ; cm.
Includes bibliographical references and index.
ISBN 978-1-84310-615-9 (pbk. : alk. paper) 1. Psychotherapist and patient. 2. Psychothera-
pists--Psychology. 3. Alternative medicine specialists--Psychology. I. Title.
[DNLM: 1. Professional-Patient Relations. 2. Psychotherapy--methods. 3. Complementary Thera-
pies--psychology. 4. Professional Role. WM 420 F794r 2008]
RC480.8.F675 2008
616.89'14--dc22
2007025972

British Library Cataloguing in Publication Data
A CIP catalogue record for this book is available from the British Library

ISBN 978 1 84310 615 9

Printed and bound in Great Britain by
Athenaeum Press, Gateshead, Tyne and Wear

Relating to Clients

of related interest

Counsellors in Health Settings
Edited by Kim Etherington
Foreword by Tim Bond
ISBN 978 1 85302 938 7

Health, the Individual, and Integrated Medicine
Revisiting an Aesthetic of Health Care
David Aldridge
ISBN 978 1 84310 232 8

Communication Skills in Practice
A Practical Guide for Health Professionals
Diana Williams
ISBN 978 1 85302 232 6

Complementary Therapies in Context
The Psychology of Healing
Helen Graham
ISBN 978 1 85302 640 9

Dyslexia and Alternative Therapies
Maria Chivers
ISBN 978 1 84310 378 3
JKP Essentials series

Understanding Controversial Therapies for Children with Autism,
Attention Deficit Disorder, and Other Learning Disabilities
Lisa A. Kurtz
978 1 84310 864 1
JKP Essentials series

Contents

Introduction

I am a psychotherapist and a complementary therapist, practising massage and craniosacral therapy. Over the years I've received shiatsu, acupuncture, homeopathy, osteopathy, physiotherapy, sports and Thai massage, Reiki and other kinds of healing, reflexology and kinesiology, trained as a healer, participated in numerous personal growth workshops and had two personal therapies, each several years long. In my practice I work with some people within a traditional psychotherapy framework; we sit opposite each other and talk, and our physical contact is limited to a formal handshake on first meeting, and, maybe, a hug when we part. With other people I'm a massage therapist and our business is very much concerned with the body, and a naked body at that, one that I'm expected to stroke, squeeze, pummel and manipulate to relieve pain, tension or stress levels. As a craniosacral therapist I also make contact with the body but gently, subtly and with different intention.

As the years go by I've become more aware of the different hats that I wear according to which therapy I'm practising. Not just hats; I wear completely different clothes – a uniform of white T-shirt and navy or black cotton trousers for massage and my own clothes for anything else. But the person I present to the client varies. For example, with a psychotherapy client I disclose very little about my personal life, because our work is to do with the client's life, problems and inner world and too much information from me would interfere. But with a massage client I might talk about my holidays, say, or a new café on the high street. A little social conversation oils the wheels of the relationship and my aim is to help the client relax with me. The sort of relationship I have with psychotherapy clients and physical therapy clients is very different. With the former group I'm consciously using the relationship as part of the work, noticing my reactions, looking for ways that the client might be using me and for patterns in the way they relate to me. But I also use these skills with complementary therapy clients too, often automatically since they are such a part of my professional self that I'm not aware of using them. My background as a psychotherapist gives me an understanding and awareness of the dynamics of the therapeutic relationship that is, by now, second nature. I don't have to think about how this knowledge intuitively informs how I relate to all the clients, students and supervisees that I work with.

While researching my proposal for this book, I interviewed five psychotherapists, who have been trained to understand the importance of the therapeutic relationship, about their personal experiences with complementary and alternative medicine (CAM) practitioners. The therapies they mentioned were massage, homeopathy, osteopathy and acupuncture. One question, based on my belief that complementary therapists didn't always understand the importance of the interactions between themselves and their clients, was to ask if they, the psychotherapists I interviewed, had had any personal experiences of misunderstandings, or discomfort, or insensitivity when visiting a complementary therapist, that might be understood to stem from inadequate training in this area. Without exception, all had examples, which came to mind straight away, of experiences involving intrusive or disrespectful behaviours, which led to feeling unsafe with the practitioner. No fewer than four people in my sample had been disturbed when osteopaths took phone calls during their treatments, and, in one case, discussed other clients. Knowing that the room wasn't soundproof and the conversation could be overheard had prevented one person from talking easily to a homeopath. Others mentioned other people actually coming into the room during a treatment. The most invasive experience was that of a woman with a history of abuse, who asked a massage practitioner to avoid working on specific parts of her body and went into shock when her request was ignored. Also mentioned were therapists, one a massage practitioner, one an acupuncturist, who were verbally invasive, either talking about their own issues or asking questions and then talking over the answer. Three interviewees mentioned the discomfort of being treated as an object, or a thing, during sessions when basic human contact seemed to be missing.

It is possible that my interviewees, being practised in the art of relationship within a therapeutic context, may be more sensitised than others to disruptions in the flow than other clients. However, much of their evidence points to a lack of appreciation among the complementary therapists they had visited that small details, like privacy, listening without interrupting and making sure that a treatment session isn't interrupted, are important.

The impetus behind this book arose from a growing awareness of the need to translate material from psychotherapy, which has developed a vast body of theoretical knowledge and beliefs about good practice to do with the therapeutic relationship, into a language that the complementary therapist could understand, and to offer ideas that translate easily into any therapeutic relationship, no matter what discipline the practitioner comes from. This is part of a growing exchange between the worlds of the talking and the body-based therapies. Psychotherapy is taking on board the body, having been for over a hundred years the 'talking cure' that was concerned with thoughts and feelings in an abstract sense. The current expansion of research findings linking emotions with particular neurochemicals, emotional behaviour with neural pathways in the brain, trauma and post-traumatic stress responses to alterations in the normal functioning of the autonomic nervous system is causing ripples of interest in the psychotherapy world and attempts to bridge the gap between mind and body. The old paradigm that declared them to be separate entities — even though the debate about the existence or location of mind, or consciousness, which has absorbed philosophers, scientists and religions for centuries, has never been solved — is giving way to a new one, a paradigm that sees not only mind and body as part of the same, but sees each one of us as interconnected, and, further than that, sees the whole universe as connected and each individual, each living being, each living cell as part of a coherent functioning whole, pulsing with life…

The therapeutic relationship is about what happens between two people, who are interconnected on a spiritual, energetic, mental, emotional and physical level. One of them has the loose title of 'healer, therapist, doctor, practitioner, guide'; the other can be called the 'patient, client, seeker, sufferer'. These terms suggest an imbalance, which is indeed so. One person has skill, expertise and knowledge; the other has a problem that causes suffering. But on another level, both are experts and both suffer. The concept of the wounded healer has powerful currency. How many of us came into the profession we now find ourselves in because of our own ills? Therapist and client are in it together, and share a mutual reality during the session. As the Buddhists say, we are mutually co-arising. My client learns from me and I from him.

But when I am the one in possession of the label healer, therapist or practitioner, I am also the one responsible for the therapeutic relationship. Not for dictating what will happen, but for establishing the boundaries and holding the space. Not for deciding what is in the client's interest but for negotiating and communicating clearly about possible outcomes. I'm responsible for my health and well being, my fitness to practise and ability to use myself as a resource in the work. I'm responsible for ensuring that I have good listening and communications skills. It's my job to have thought about power and sex in the therapeutic relation and how I use touch with my clients.

It is hoped that this book will fill the gap, by providing information, theory, some research and exercises for the reader to try to add a practical dimension to the learning. Although many of the exercises derive from the world of psychotherapy, the intention is not to turn the complementary therapist into a psychotherapist, but instead to share helpful material.

The exercises in the book

Do our thoughts affect others? Some of the exercises in this book ask you to own up to negative thoughts and feelings, and, what's more, suggest that you may have some of these towards the very people that you work with, the ones you are supposed to care for and help.

The business of psychotherapy involves a lot of this kind of stuff, talking about the unacceptable, the shameful or embarrassing aspects of ourselves. It involves exploring the darker sides of our nature. It rakes over the past, exposing the people or events that have been harmful. Psychotherapy allows the wicked thoughts, the murderous fantasies, the desires for revenge and the secret passions to be named. There's an awful lot of negative thinking and destructive emoting goes on in psychotherapists' treatment rooms in the name of healing.

The intention of this sort of work isn't to blame or hurt people from the client's past or to keep negative memory alive, or to legitimise feelings of victimhood (I had a terrible upbringing therefore the world must look after me and I can't be held responsible for my actions) but to acknowledge thoughts and feelings and release them. Freud is famous for saying that the goal of therapy is to convert neurotic misery into ordinary unhappiness. If we can accept that constant happiness is an unrealistic ideal, it's easier to tolerate life's ups and downs for what they are. The only thing we can ever know for sure is that everything changes. There's a level at which we have to accept that we do not live in a perfect world where people smile at each other all the time and everyone is healthy, housed and happy. The serenity prayer used in 12-step programmes all over the world points to this when it says:

> God, grant me the serenity to accept the things that I cannot change
> Courage to change the things that I can
> And wisdom to know the difference.
>
> (Niebuhr 1986, p.87)

In *Teachings on Love* (1998) the Buddhist teacher Thich Nhat Hanh writes 'The first step in dealing with our unconscious internal formations is to try to bring them into consciousness.' Internal formations are the knots of misunderstanding accompanied by negative emotions that form when we are subject to an unpleasant event. Using breathing, mindfulness meditation and self observation, eventually, he says, we come to know and make peace with these formations.

You may have treated people with a cancer diagnosis. The cancer, until it began to produce symptoms or was detected by regular screening, was a destructive force hidden in the tissues. If such a growth is ignored there's a likelihood that it will grow, invade or compress other tissues, cause more damage and possibly bring about the death of the body it inhabits. Destructive thoughts don't kill people, but they do create the sort of neurochemicals associated with anxiety or depression and too many of those in the system over a long period can contribute to poor physical health. Your client with cancer may have had surgery, chemo or radiotherapy to remove the cancer. On the whole, there's an agreement that the body is better off without this sort of 'bad' stuff. So too for cancerous thinking, the sort that takes seed and spreads – the body is better off without it. In both cases, the first step is to make visible that which has been hidden and acknowledge its presence. The next is to have a look at it and decide what is to be done. Then the letting go/getting rid of process, together with coming to terms with the effect of the 'bad' stuff, how things could have been different, what might have created it, and finally moving to a resolution and getting on with life.

The aim of all healing is to face, acknowledge, mourn, accept, and move on. And this is the intention with these exercises. Complementary therapists aren't merely nice, caring, wonderful people. Like all other human beings we get impatient, frustrated, dislike certain sorts of people and the exercises invite you to explore some of these aspects of yourself. A friend of mine says to himself, when he finds himself being critical (or whatever negative thought has popped into his awareness), 'Oh hello, little critical thought. What have you got to tell me today?' He actually welcomes his negative thoughts for what he can learn about himself from them. You won't harm your clients if you allow yourself to think difficult thoughts about them, but you might learn something about yourself and become an even better practitioner than you are already.

Terminology

There are different words in common use to describe the person who is offering and the person who has come for treatment. In the psychotherapeutic world, we have analysts, psychotherapists (often shortened to therapist) and counsellors. The person on the receiving end of psychoanalysis is the analysand or the patient, and of most other psychotherapies, the client. In the complementary therapy world we have acupuncturists, masseurs, chiropractors, homeopaths, teachers of Alexander technique, colour healers, Reiki masters, Feldenkrais practitioners, craniosacral therapists, traditional Chinese medicine (TCM) practitioners, kinesiologists, iridologists, reflexologists, naturopaths, zero balancers, to name but a few. General names for this group are complementary therapists or CAM practitioners.

The majority of complementary therapists work in private practice and the people they treat pay for their services: this financial aspect to the relationship is reflected in the use of the term client. Homeopaths are the exception, calling the people they treat patients, possibly because it was practised by the medical establishment and was, briefly, mainstream during the late nineteenth and early twentieth centuries. Osteopaths working in the National Health Service (NHS) use the term patients, but tend to use clients in private practice.

Throughout the book, I'll use the term client for the receiver, psychotherapist for practitioner of the talking therapies and practitioner or complementary therapist for the other.

Although the majority of practitioners and users of complementary therapies tend to be women, I've tried to avoid any gender bias by alternating the pronouns she and he throughout the text.

All case material used in this book is either fictitious or, where drawn from real life, substantially altered so as to preserve confidentiality.

1

What is the Professional Therapeutic Relationship?

A woman walks through a field, a garden, a park. She's in a hurry on her way to work, she's distracted by a message on her phone, she's weeping because her lover has left, she's running to collect her child, she's running away from her past. She walks and sees nothing.

A woman walks slowly though a field, a garden, a park. The air is sharp and tinged with leaves burning, the air is warm and rose scented, the air is moist and smells of earth after rain. The grass is neatly mowed, the grass is long and yellowing and waves in the breeze, the grass is fresh green dotted with daisies. The woman names the flowers to herself: buttercup, cow parsley, ragged robin, begonia, petunia, busy lizzie. She walks and is mindful.

A woman walks through a field, a garden, a park. Every leaf, blade of grass and petal is vibrating with life, colours intensely vivid, the air dancing with spirits and singing. Energy streams through her and around her, the woman and the plants and the earth, connected in a living, pulsing web. For a moment, the woman walks and the veil between the worlds is lifted.

There are many ways of being in the world. There are many ways of relating to our fellow human beings. The more we can be present and mindful and aware, the more richness and potential there is to touch another's soul and to let ourselves be touched. If you've ever been involved in an intense group activity you might have come across that sense of really meeting the others who were on the journey with you. We are introduced to someone at a party, we chat for five minutes and then say 'Nice to meet you'. But we didn't, not really, meet that person, or let ourselves be met, not our raw, strange, wonderful and quite unique selves. We let others see the version that's been modified for public consumption. In the descriptions above, the woman's awareness of her surroundings ranged from nearly oblivious to totally interactional. In a similar way, we, as complementary health professionals, can be ignorant of or attentive to the framework within which we relate to the people we work with.

Maybe it helps to define the purpose of this book if we consider the different types of relationship that can exist between two people, relationships that we might define as therapeutic. Let's begin by thinking about the professional and the therapeutic aspects. At its most basic, the professional relationship is one in which one person is qualified to offer particular services to another, and is remunerated for this in some way. There is a clear contractual element, and the relationship takes place within a specific context such as an office, a treatment room, a website or wherever the professional works. It is time limited, so when the services are no longer required, the professional relationship ends. This description applies to lawyers, homeopaths, doctors, plumbers, architects, garage mechanics and many others.

The therapeutic relationship exists when one person offers help, support or caring to another person in need. At its most informal level, a therapeutic relationship exists when a mother washes and puts a plaster on her child's grazed knee, or when someone offers a shoulder massage to a stressed friend, or an elderly person who's fallen in the street is helped by a passer by. The helper may or may not be qualified to do so, the relationship may be a familial one or between two strangers, and the services offered may not be reciprocated. There is no contract.

A professional therapeutic relationship exists whenever two (or more, if the one who needs healing is a child or an adult needing an advocate or interpreter) people meet, and one has skills and expertise which the other wants to alleviate suffering, or, for many people who consult CAM practitioners, to maintain levels of health and well being. The relationship is contractual, governed by legal, professional and ethical guidelines and the practitioner is remunerated for her services. The professional therapeutic relationship takes place within a particular setting such as a treatment room, a clinic, a hospital, a health centre or the client's own home. The professional therapeutic relationship ends when the services are no longer required, but there may be exceptions to this, which we'll consider later.

Therapeutic relationship as treatment only

What happens within the professional therapeutic relationship? At its most basic, there's the setting, an exchange of money, a professional, a client and the treatment. In some contexts the focus is entirely on the treatment. If you have been to Turkey you may, like me, have been to a Turkish bath or hammam and had the wonderful experience of lying on a marble slab, covered with rose-scented lather, pummelled and rinsed down. For me, this was definitely a therapeutic experience and I felt great afterwards, and it was also a professional one (I asked – the masseur was qualified) but the interaction between us was minimal, limited to gestures on his part – come here, lie down, turn over, we're finished. I wouldn't have recognised him if I'd passed him in the street an hour later. Another therapeutic experience I've had which focused entirely on the treatment was using flotation tanks. There was a person involved, who asked if I was pregnant, had high blood pressure or was taking medication, showed me what to do, and waited somewhere outside to let me out if I pushed the panic button and who turned off the music and turned on the lights when my session was over. My body felt soft and relaxed, as if I'd had a massage without being touched. The therapeutic relationship was minimal but I had had a therapeutic treatment.

An image of this level of professional therapeutic relationship would look like this:

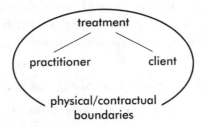

Figure 1.1 Therapeutic relationship as treatment only

Therapeutic relationship with interpersonal skills

To move on to the next level of complexity, we have the sort of relationship that is professional and therapeutic, and there is a treatment involving the skills and expertise of the practitioner, and there is something more that has a definite effect on the outcome. This additional factor is the relationship between the practitioner and client. When I taught professional massage training, there was an exercise I used to demonstrate the importance of the practitioner's attitude and behaviour during an initial consultation. I'd role-play with a willing accomplice how not to do a good consultation. It would go something like this:

> The 'practitioner' (me) is sitting with her feet up on the treatment couch talking on her mobile phone and eating an apple. There's a knock on the door. It's the 'client'.
>
> Practitioner calls out, without moving, 'Come in, I'm on the phone. Sit down, be with you in a minute.'
>
> The client enters, looks round for somewhere to sit and, seeing the only other chair holds a pile of towels, puts them on the floor before sitting down.
>
> Practitioner finishes her call and says 'That was my friend; we're meeting up after work and were trying to decide where to eat. Don't suppose you know any good bars in town? No, never mind. OK now, you want a massage, right? What for?'

Client looks bemused.

Before she can answer, practitioner rushes on, 'Relaxation? Sore shoulders? Strained something? Come on, we haven't got all day.'

Client is by now looking a little upset, but manages to say that she's been feeling a little stressed lately.

Practitioner, still with her feet on the table: 'Stress hum. Work deadlines, moving house or your mother died? Don't worry, I'm well known for my stress expertise. OK, now some medical information. What's wrong with you?'

Client hesitates.

Practitioner continues, 'Oh you look fine to me. No aches and pains? OK then, just take all your clothes off and lie down on the couch. I'll call my next client to confirm her appointment while you do that.'

Client, looking very tearful, gets up and walks out of the room.

And then, when the laughing stopped, we'd all work out where this 'practitioner' was going wrong and, from this, identify elements of good practice in establishing a working relationship with a client. The list would look like this:

- clear boundaries between personal and professional

- being able to make a clear contract with the client

- being prepared

- good listening skills

- communicating clearly and simply

- empathy

- focusing on the client

- and, in the case of the 'practitioner' above, being polite.

So now we have a professional therapeutic relationship where the treatment and the relationship both have an impact on the eventual outcome. A visual image would look like this:

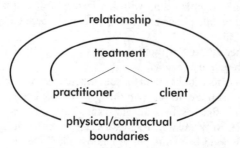

Figure 1.2 Therapeutic relationship as treatment influenced by practitioner – client relationship contained within professional boundaries

Some people are very good at relating to others, and others struggle. Some can talk with ease, others are pretty inarticulate. Some are confident, others are shy. For some, good listening is second nature while others can't recall what someone said two minutes ago. Some attune to others' emotional states without even knowing that they are doing it, while others do anything to avoid feelings. But whatever a person's strengths and weaknesses in this area, interpersonal skills can be improved. We can learn to communicate simply, or to listen well, or to keep good boundaries. The skills involved in establishing and maintaining good practitioner–client relationships are relevant to practitioners of all kinds of complementary therapies, from Reiki to Rolfing, homeopathy to herbalism, iridology to Indian head massage. And if interpersonal skills are as important as the treatment, why not do everything we can to use them consciously and improve our weaknesses?

Self awareness is another factor that helps us to relate smoothly to others. For example, it helps to be aware of our beliefs and accompanying feelings about people who are different from us. It helps to have explored the reasons why we came into a helping profession, so that we are clear about our hidden as well as our conscious motivation for being a complementary therapist. Our families are our first teachers when it comes to interpersonal relating and, however hard they tried, there were bound to have been mistakes. It helps to have explored the rules you internalised as a child and to have an awareness of problematic relationships and how that affected you.

And for most practitioners, most of the time, with most clients, good interpersonal skills and self awareness are sufficient. But there are occasions when difficulties arise, we feel out of our depth, are puzzled by client's reactions, are puzzled by our own feelings and just can't make out what is going on. Have you ever looked at your client list for the day and felt dread at seeing someone's name, even though you know he is a perfectly pleasant person? Or felt unaccountably hungry after seeing another client even though you just had lunch? Or experienced fuzziness and found it hard to think clearly when talking to another? This brings us to yet another level of the professional therapeutic relationship, one that the psychotherapists understand.

The therapeutic aspect of the relationship itself

There are many different schools of psychotherapy and counselling, just as there are many different kinds of complementary therapies. On the whole, and unlike complementary therapies, practitioners of most schools tend to emphasise the relationship rather than the treatment aspect of the work. The psychoanalytic schools of psychotherapy work entirely with the relationship between therapist and client – this is the treatment. There are also types that don't worry much at all about the relationship, notably the cognitive and behavioural therapies, which focus on the treatment, setting clear objective goals and planning strategies to achieve them. With the relationship foreground in the healing, the treatment, which in psychotherapy terms means the theoretical models about the mind and any tools that the therapists might use, takes on far less importance. Tools, for a psychotherapist, might be making what are called interpretations, which means saying just the right thing at the right moment to create a shift in the client's understanding or awareness. Another tool is dream interpretation. Tools used by both psychotherapists and some CAM practitioners are visualisation, breath work or writing or drawing exercises.

In this sort of professional therapeutic relationship, we still have the boundaries, the practitioner and his or her use of interpersonal skills and self awareness, the treatment and the client. But we also have everything else that both parties are bringing to the relationship, some of which is conscious and spoken (Client to acupuncturist: 'I'm a bit anxious about the needles. Will they hurt?') and some of which is conscious but not spoken (reflexologist thinking about client: 'You do look just like my horrible aunty Janet'). And then there is all the material that isn't particularly conscious at all, such as our history as a CAM practitioner, and the client's history as a client. And all our personal history and all of the client's. Values, attitudes, prejudices, cultural background, gender and sexual orientation, religious and spiritual beliefs and the stuff that some people call our 'baggage', the unhealed wounds from the past, it's as if all of this material is floating around inside the therapeutic relationship. The client's relationship with her mother bumps up against the practitioner in the here and now. A large male client activates the practitioner's fears about large men. The unmet need to be loved raises its head and thinks, 'Maybe this time...?'

All sorts of things can occur at this level of the professional therapeutic relationship. It's a bit like walking into an enchanted forest, where nothing is quite as it seems and the rules of ordinary life are suspended and patience is required to see what will happen next. There's a lot of analogy, symbolism and magic. And psychotherapists are trained to deal with this world. And we, CAM practitioners, are not, so it isn't our job to be able to work in this way, and I have no intention of turning complementary therapists into psychotherapists, but I do think, however, that there are some useful things that we can learn from our colleagues in the talking therapy field. There are ways of describing processes that occur, not just in a therapeutic context but also in any sort of relationship. Just as body workers have a map in their mind of the underlying tissues and organs which informs how they make sense of the information obtained through palpation, and TCM practitioners have an internal map of the meridians which enables them to know where energy might be stagnating, so psychotherapists have maps to describe, for example, how one person can project aspects of himself onto another, or how a person internalises (takes in) parts of another. Or how a client might use a therapeutic relationship to provide an aspect of experience that was missing in her early life. When these sorts of processes are evoked in a professional therapeutic relationship, things can seem uncomfortable, confusing or even disturbing for the practitioner, and this is where a little understanding can help. In later sections of the book I explain these processes and offer tools for the use of the practitioner to help her understand her own part of the process. And I would emphasise that, no matter how good we become at being our own inner supervisor, professional help and support from an experienced (external!) supervisor is essential to good practice.

A visual image of this level of professional therapeutic relationship would look something like this:

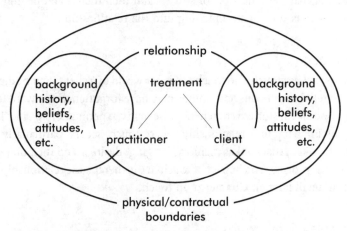

Figure 1.3 Therapeutic relationship that acknowledges the part played by the practitioner – client relationship in the overall treatment

Unconscious process of the sort just mentioned is unlikely to be an important feature in the majority of practitioner–client interactions for the complementary health professional, but there are certain conditions that, I believe, might make it more likely.

Length of relationship

The longer a professional therapeutic relationship continues, the more likely it is that unconscious processes will be present, for both practitioner and client.

In a long-term relationship, the practitioner may get to know a lot about the client's personal life, and for both people, an attachment can develop.

Intimacy of information shared

Some complementary therapies work more deliberately with the client's emotional life than others, homeopathy being a good example. The more a person is asked to share personal details, the more the client's inner world will be stirred up. She may find herself talking about things that she hasn't told anyone else. Questions about the onset of a condition, the symptoms and even the client's understanding about why this might be happening to her now are relatively objective. Questions about her likes and dislikes reach a bit further in, about her relationships, self esteem or perspective on life further still and asking about trauma or abuse can touch a very deep place. The practitioner who asks very personal questions shows an interest usually only experienced with close friends and partners, if then. This can make a person feel special – or invaded but that's another sort of story – and then there's an opening for all the unconscious stuff to start moving into the relationship.

Use of touch

Therapies that use touch also touch the inner world of a client. Our bodies have stories to tell that our conscious minds may have forgotten or not want to hear. When a body with stories is touched it's been given permission to talk. There's a level of intimacy in a relationship where touch occurs, particularly if the receiver is naked, that evokes memory, longing, desire…and the potential for unconscious process. The impact of touch in the therapeutic relationship is discussed in detail later, in Chapter 6 on touch.

Vulnerable client groups

There are certain client groups that are more likely to evoke unconscious process in the practitioner. People with learning disability, with mental health problems and people in recovery from alcohol or substance abuse, those who are terminally ill, people with severe eating disorders, those who've been raped, abused or tortured, all of these can evoke beliefs, fears and anxieties about difference, incapacity, madness and dying. Until we are confronted, many of us prefer not to have to think about such things.

And for many in the client groups mentioned above, the ability to 'be adult' or to stay present in here-and-now reality may be compromised. Most of us are able to act as adults most of the time. When we say 'I really lost it' we're referring to an occasion when our normal adult functioning slipped and we got into a rage, started crying helplessly or behaved in a manner inappropriate to the situation. Even when this sort of thing happens, there's usually a part of ourselves looking on, uninvolved, just witnessing. But for some people this isn't possible. For others, the ability to stay in present reality may be hard. When a client's process is activated, the practitioner needs particular skills to deal with this.

Models of the therapeutic relationship
Treatment or relationship

Stone and Katz, writing for CAM practitioners in *Perspectives on Complementary and Alternative Medicine* (2005), describe a range of relationship possibilities, all of which have at their core one person who offers and another who needs healing. A therapeutic relationship exists whenever two (or more, if the one who needs healing is a child or an adult needing an advocate or interpreter) people meet, and one has skills and expertise that the other wants to alleviate suffering. Another way of understanding is that the therapeutic relationship consists of the treatment itself plus the relationship or rapport that builds up over several consultations between practitioner and client. Then there is the view that the main component in the healing is the relationship itself with the treatment as secondary importance. This view is based on the belief that people sometimes choose to see a CAM practitioner because they offer better attention and interest, treat clients as individuals rather than a bundle of symptoms and take the context of their illness into account, unlike their counterparts in traditional medicine. However, as Stone and Katz point out, there is a move within this field away from a mechanistic view towards a more biosocial one that places the patient and her illness in the wider context of her whole life. Government initiatives require health carers to listen to patients' perceptions of their illness and to encourage them to take some responsibility for their treatment. They also quote findings from a study by Kelner in Canada who compared patients' relationships with their general practitioners (GPs) to those they had with CAM practitioners (Kelner 2000, quoted in Lee-Treweek 2005). The rapport with GPs, their willingness to listen, to explain what they were doing and to involve patients in decisions was found to be more or less the same as in the CAM practitioner–patient relationship.

The sliding scale model

Kelner (2000) offers a sliding scale model of the therapeutic relationship:

1. The paternalistic relationship where both parties involved assume that the practitioner knows best and takes full responsibility for

decisions about the client's care, and all the client has to do is follow the advice he is given.

2. The mutual relationship based on listening and negotiation, where both parties have a say in decisions about treatment and the client takes some responsibility for his own healing.

3. The user-dominated model, based on the notion of the user as a consumer of services with the power to pick and choose his practitioner and his therapy.

Key features of the CAM therapeutic relationship

Mitchell and Cormack (1998), also writing about the therapeutic relationship for CAM practitioners, describe its key features:

1. CAM is holistic and assumes an interconnection of mind, body and spirit. Although few practitioners would claim to work with each of these levels, there is an understanding that healing on one level will have beneficial impact on the others too.

2. Each person is assessed as an individual and treatment tailored to the person. Symptoms are understood in the context of the whole body, the person's social situation, and recent life events.

3. There is an emphasis on treating chronic disorders.

4. There is relatively low risk of side effects.

5. Users are expected to help themselves.

6. There's an emphasis on the user's perspective.

7. A broad definition of health is used.

In their book they emphasise the role of the relationship as a key element in the process of change and highlight the importance of the qualities of warmth, empathy, trust, respect and mutuality in the practitioner.

From a psychotherapeutic perspective

Petruska Clarkson, writing for counsellors and psychotherapists in her book *The Therapeutic Relationship* (1995), describes five modes of relating within the therapeutic relationship. These are not exclusive and, at different times in the course of one therapeutic relationship, all of them could be present, maybe overlapping, maybe consecutively. For example, the working alliance refers to the phase where the relationship is just being established and both parties are discovering if they can work together, so this kind of interaction would be more common in the beginning.

The working alliance

In order for two people to work well together, there has to be an agreement as to the nature of their task and how they are going to arrive at their goals. There has to be an element of trust between them and a willingness to cooperate. In the complementary therapy relationship the working alliance depends on how well the initial contract is managed, the interpersonal skills of the practitioner and personal factors of both people such as age, gender and cultural background. The client's expectations of what a therapist should be like, and the match or mismatch with her expectations may affect the alliance. For example, as Petruska Clarkson suggests, a businessman in a suit may find it hard to believe that a young woman in a tracksuit can help him. The client's previous experience of health-care professionals, or authority figures in general, will have some bearing on her ability to trust and enter into a good alliance. To some extent this can be ascertained by asking, when taking details about the client's doctor, consultant or previous CAM therapists, how well she got on with them.

The real relationship

Sometimes called the person-to-person relationship, the real relationship, like Kelner's mutual relationship, involves a two-way communication and a willingness on the part of the practitioner to put aside his professional role and be present as a human being, to allow himself to be affected by and fully present with his client in the here and now, and able to admit his fallibility. Although this sounds like an ideal way to relate, it is fraught with potential danger. The practitioner can't just 'be himself' if, for example, he has a bad hangover, the client reminds him of an overbearing aunt or he finds the client's accent unbearably funny. His 'real' responses must be contained, having no useful place in the therapeutic relationship. Sharing personal experience can be a very therapeutic part of a person-to-person relationship, but the practitioner needs to be sensitive to the risk of intruding his own material into the session. (See the section on disclosure in Chapter 3, p.76)

The transference–countertransference relationship

This mode of relationship, first described by Freud and elaborated by subsequent generations of psychoanalysts, is now generally accepted by most schools of psychotherapy as a common occurrence in a therapeutic relationship, where it can exist alongside a working alliance, and/or a real relationship. I will describe the transference–countertransference relationship in greater detail later on, as well as how to recognise it when it occurs and offer tools for understanding the dynamics.

The reparative relationship

In psychotherapy this usually refers to a relationship where the therapist deliberately provides the sorts of experiences which were missing during the client's early life, such as attuning to her inner world, helping her in order to correct, for want of a better term, mistakes. This requires knowledge of childhood development, an acceptance that child-rearing norms are based on white middle-class values and are not universal and an ability to deal with regression when it happens.

Regression is a phenomenon that can happen in everyday life as well as within a therapeutic relationship, and is not uncommon. Who has not at some point suddenly felt as if they were no longer a functioning adult but a small child? Or found themselves reliving the thoughts and feelings of a past trauma as if it were happening in the present? Some psychotherapies encourage regression as a means of reliving and reworking wounding experiences from the past, with more or less emphasis on an adult part of the client, a witness, staying present. Regressive moments can occur spontaneously in any therapeutic relationship including the CAM practitioner–client one, but I would hazard a guess that this would be more likely in therapies where a long-term relationship may develop and those where a lot of personal information is divulged, such as homeopathy, or in therapies that use touch, particularly nurturing rather than diagnostic touch. Survivors of sexual or physical abuse in childhood may choose nurturing body therapies such as aromatherapy or massage as a means of consciously trying to have a reparative experience of touch and regression may occur as part of the explorative journey.

The transpersonal

The last of Petruska Clarkson's modes of therapeutic relationship, the transpersonal, is the hardest to define and probably the one that happens in rare moments rather than as an ongoing way of relating between practitioner and client. The transpersonal refers to the spiritual, mysterious, numinous, religious, to the times which have a different quality from ordinary day-to-day experience, which some describe as altered states of consciousness. Both practitioner and client may have strong spiritual beliefs but this doesn't mean that the transpersonal will occur in their working relationship, and, on the other hand, two agnostics may find themselves sharing an out of the ordinary moment. I once watched a craniosacral therapy teacher demonstrating to a group. He sat at the head of the woman who had been chosen and gently cradled her skull in his hands and waited. The silence and stillness in the room deepened. No one moved. After a while the atmosphere shifted perceptibly and it was as if a new force had entered the room, one that seemed to open my heart centre. I had tears running down my face and, looking round the group, saw I wasn't the only person to have been touched in this way. This was a transpersonal moment.

Working with the spiritual dimension

There's a major difference here between psychotherapy and complementary therapy, namely that, with a few exceptions, psychotherapy deals with the secular rather than the spiritual, and many, but not all, complementary therapies have foundations in an energetic, non-material belief system. Core process therapy and psychosynthesis are two talking therapies with a spiritual basis and a person seeking a psychotherapist who includes a spiritual dimension in the work may well choose from one of these schools. Counsellors working with the bereaved, or those facing death, may well explore ideas about dying and what happens afterwards, but apart from these situations, it is generally considered good practice by psychotherapists and counsellors to avoid introducing ideas about the transpersonal into the work, certainly to never impose their own belief systems on clients, and to wait until the subject is introduced by the client.

CAM practitioners who work with a therapy with an energetic/spiritual base have a problem when it comes to explaining to new clients how their therapy works. Although use of the concept of 'energy' is becoming more commonplace, not everyone understands it (do we, using it as freely as we do?) and to give a description that some might find too 'wafty' leads to the danger of alienating and losing clients. As service providers we have a responsibility to be clear what it is we're offering.

A healer is asked what she will do to treat a painful arthritic knee. Consider these two possible explanations.

> I'll sit quietly for a while before I put my hands on your body, and let my mind settle down. Then I'll hold your knee and let the heat from my hands soften and relax the tissues that have tightened up around the joint in response to the pain that you're feeling.

> Before I start I'll shut my eyes and ask my guides and the angels to be present. Then I'll wrap us both up in white light. When I put my hands on your knee

I'll surrender to the flow of energy from the source and allow myself to become a channel, and that energy will go where it needs in your body.

Both versions are 'true' descriptions but use different frameworks to describe the treatment. If you were a person unfamiliar with complementary therapy, which version do you think would sound more reassuring? Do you think the healer using the second version is imposing her belief system on the client?

When it comes to talking about the spiritual or the transpersonal, the practitioner might consider the following guidelines:

- Be sensitive to the client's openness to ideas about energy or the spiritual dimension.

- Communicate the energetic basis of your treatment as simply as you can, with confidence.

- If possible, also give an explanation in familiar medical terms, relating it to anatomy and physiology.

- Don't impose an energy-only rationale. Have respect for other models.

Why does the therapeutic relationship matter to complementary therapists?

Very little is taught about the therapeutic relationship, its importance and how to create effective ones, on complementary therapy trainings. Research shows that the most important factor in a successful psychotherapy treatment is the relationship between the therapist and the client, not the school or model of counselling or psychotherapy used. If these findings are translatable to complementary therapy, then it could mean that the relationship with an individual CAM practitioner is as important as the therapy she or he practises. One such piece of research was carried out in 1999 by Mark Hubble, Barry Duncan and Scott Miller, for the American Psychological Association. They looked at the factors that make for a successful psychotherapy and describe their findings in a book called *Heart and Soul of Change: What Works in Therapy*. The single most important factor, contributing to 40 per cent of a successful outcome, was the client himself and what he brought to the relationship, including his strengths, support network, previous life experience and an ability to share in the responsibility for change. The type of therapy practised was of comparatively little importance, accounting for only 15 per cent of the outcome. Of far greater importance were the human factors and the nature of the relationship which included the therapist's empathy, acceptance, affirmation, encouragement.

Both people need to believe that the therapy will work. Hope, placebo and expectancy contributed 15 per cent to a good outcome. They concluded that 'research strongly suggests that what clients find helpful in therapy has little to do with the techniques that the therapists find so important…the most helpful factor was having the time and a place to focus on themselves and talk' (p.105).

However sometimes a particular treatment is recommended, suggesting that the interpersonal relationship is not that important a factor. Lord Layard's report (2006) recommends cognitive behavioural therapy (CBT) rather than any other kind of psychological therapy for treatment of anxiety and depression by the National Health Service. There are several good reasons for this, which include the fact that CBT is, as the name suggests, a behavioural therapy, involving the establishment of a clear objective treatment goal for the client. It is far easier to measure, say, ability to travel three steps on the underground, in a person with acute travel phobia, then to measure success in a client with repeated abandonment issues from childhood and a history of depression, who finds intimate relationship difficulty. Or someone who is facing death from a terminal illness, or an asylum seeker who is not only living in an unfamiliar culture, but has witnessed his family murdered.

CBT does have a high success rate, but another element to take into account is that practitioners can be selective about who they choose to treat. The client must be motivated and willing to do the homework required alongside the sessions. Clients who aren't prepared to participate fully may not be accepted. So CBT is a highly successful therapy, but with a selected client group, and certain issues.

Good and bad experiences of health-care professionals

While researching my proposal for this book, I met with four colleagues (one practised massage, one reflexology, one psychotherapy and one psychotherapeutical body work) to talk about the therapeutic relationship. We began by recalling the worst and the best experiences we'd had with a health-care professional, as a way to begin thinking about good practice. The first thing to emerge was how much easier it was to remember the bad times, in vivid detail, often with remnants of the original emotional charge. So, for example, Jo's voice shook with anger when she talked about her experience with a dentist who, on seeing her nervously clasped hands in her lap as she lay supine, waiting for the pain to begin, had grabbed the offending hands, raised then in the air, shouting 'For Christ's sake, relax!' Insulting words or behaviour figured in several other 'worst times' stories. Maura had suffered from a spinal disc injury in her twenties and was referred eventually to a Harley Street specialist, the best in the field. She had to wait months for an appointment, and during this period a friend recommended a chiropractor, who could see her immediately. The visit wasn't very helpful, but the worst happened when she finally had her meeting with the consultant and told the 'great man' (her words) about it. Nothing had prepared her for his tirade of anger, which left her confused, angry and very upset. Although she can't remember a word he said, she assumed it was about her audacity and stupidity in visiting a complementary therapist. This was over 20 years ago. Joyce Vetterlein, an osteopath with over 30 years' experience, talking about the public perception of her profession (private conversation 2005), recalls that, when she first started, the law making abortion legal had only just been passed, and osteopaths had a similar status to the back-street abortionists. A doctor would hand a patient a piece of paper with a name and number scribbled on it and say 'But don't tell anyone I gave you this'. Things have certainly changed since then, osteopathy being one of the few disciplines to have gained full recognition by the medical establishment.

In the group, Don and Caroline also had experiences of, not abusive, but inappropriate verbal communication. Don's severe headache had taken him to various experts, he'd had tests, he'd had a magnetic resonance imaging (MRI) scan and no cause could be found. The final doctor said 'Well, if it gets better, it doesn't matter what the cause is, does it?' At which Don lost faith in the medical establishment and took matters into his own hands, altering his diet by eliminating caffeine, wheat, dairy and sugar. The headache disappeared. In Don's case, a bad experience led to a dramatic and positive change in lifestyle. Caroline went to her general practitioner recently for removal of a little skin tag. The doctor couldn't find his scalpel, told her the tag was highly pedunculated and asked her if she'd like to take it home! As a reflexologist Caroline knew the meaning of the medical term (it means 'on a little stalk') but reflected that for someone who didn't, the comment could cause concern. And as for taking her skin tag away with her, her comment was 'Gross!'

Strangely enough, we also had complaints about over-nice professionals, who ended up being irritating or gushing. Caroline's masseuse who overused her name was a case in point, especially when she also used the wrong name. But these behaviours were nothing to those that made us feel objectified, unimportant or insulted. Bad experiences also concerned practitioners not being prepared. Caroline was seen for several sessions by a podiatrist, who never read her notes and had to be reminded why she came to see him. She felt that he wasn't really interested in her – that she was just the next one in line. This reminded me of the time I'd arrived for my massage at the home of my practitioner on the wrong day – her mistake or mine, it doesn't really matter; finding the usually warm and womblike room looking like an ordinary sitting room, and my practitioner with her hair wrapped in a towel, was upsetting to say the least. To make matters worse, I felt I had to take care of her feelings as well as my own. I extricated myself as quickly as possible and didn't go back.

The good experiences, on the other hand, either involved feeling cared for or respected as the individuals that we are, or they were effective remedies for our problems, or both. Jo recalled a professor who'd cared for her over a ten-day stay in hospital with severe pancreatic inflammation, who had been just the right mix of competent professional and caring human being. Several of us had had long-term relationships, Maura with a shiatsu practitioner, the person who did eventually clear up her back problems and me with my osteo-path. I visit Fiona once a year, if that, when my lumbar sacral disc plays up and I know that swimming, relaxation or massage won't do the trick. She always remembers me, what I've been doing and my usual skeletal weaknesses. Maybe she reads my notes before meeting me, but it doesn't matter how she remem-bers me, the fact that she does is what makes me feel good. I trust her to make me better.

Good and bad clients

When we moved on to make a list, slightly tongue in cheek, of the things that characterise a good client, some of the characteristics listed by Hubble *et al.* (1999) as important for the success of treatment were mentioned. Caroline, the reflexologist, thought that the process of healing was more effective when the client took some responsibility, thought about her condition and noticed any changes between sessions, and took on board practical advice from her practi-tioner. It helps, too, if a client can be honest about the effect of treatment. (How many just say 'That was very nice, thank you' after a massage?) Or about some-thing he may have felt uncomfortable about. Being on time, knowing when the session had finished and remembering to pay all featured prominently, as did the client who keeps coming back. A cynic might say that it's bad business to fix clients too quickly. It helps if the client appears to like us, and shows some appreciation or gratitude because it makes it easier for us to relate to them, to form a good 'working alliance', as it's known in psychotherapy. Knowing when to stop talking and the ability to let go of control were men-tioned too. At this point the two psychotherapists in the group pointed out that some of these issues would be worked with in a psychotherapeutic relation-ship, would be named and explored. Jo talked about a client, let's call her Mary, who took at least ten minutes to gather her things, put her cardigans, coat, scarf on, talking all the time, before she left the room. Jo pointed this out gently, wondering about it, and Mary explained that she always found making the transition from one space to another very difficult. That knowledge eased Jo's irritation with her client. She also decided to end the treatment ten minutes early, building in the time that Mary needed to get ready.

The non-psychotherapists in the group felt that they, too, would like to have the sort of skills that smooth out snags in the relationship. Maura said 'How do I deal with someone who throws a big wobbly? I don't know. It's my worst nightmare.' The complementary therapists talked about what they'd learned about the therapeutic relationship on their initial trainings and some said there was nothing, that the whole training had been skills based. The others said that they'd learned by watching the tutors and how they related to each other and the students, and by doing role-plays.

It is hoped that the concepts and related exercises throughout the book will provide more understanding of the therapeutic relationship and how the practitioner can use herself as a resource in the healing, and to make sense of the occasions when a relationship runs into difficulties or breaks down completely. And there is no substitute for a good supervisory relationship.

2

Practitioner Self Awareness

Part of our job as complementary therapists is to monitor and advise our clients' health and well being. Depending on our therapy, we might suggest stretching exercises, give dietary advice, recommend essential oils or vitamin supplements, prescribe Chinese herbs or explore lifestyle changes with our client. Do we practise what we preach? In this section, I want to explore the essentials of self care, first, of ourselves as human beings and, second, as human beings who work within a certain profession and have self-care needs specific to the sorts of work that we do. Professional chefs need to keep their culinary equipment in good order, artists their paints and canvases, a rusty spade is no use to a gardener and classical musicians, no matter how experienced, have to practise their scales daily. Practitioners of massage, Bowen technique, osteopathy, Feldenkrais, Rolfing and Trager work have to keep their bodies in good shape to prevent repetitive strains and back problems. Complementary therapy practitioners who use focus and intention during their treatments ideally practise techniques to clear and focus their minds. We all need to keep up to date with research and new products in our field. And we need to ensure that we don't burn out.

How well do you look after yourself? One day in a book shop, in the queue by the till, I noticed a little book on the counter, waiting there, like sweets by the supermarket checkout, to be popped in the basket. It was called *If I Really Loved Myself, I Would...* and the single sentence on each page proclaimed what the author did, having made the decision to live her life that way: eat only organic food, stop bothering what other people thought of her, throw away her too tight clothes, walk in the park every day and so on. It got me thinking about the difference between basic self maintenance and how we might do this differently if we really loved ourselves. I wondered if there was an analogy here between health defined as absence of illness, the sense of being neither ill nor really well, just ticking over, and optimum health, like the glow of well being we feel after a really enjoyable holiday. Let's start with the basics.

Self care of the body
The basics: exercise, air, food and water
EXERCISE

To keep in good shape, the current recommendations for exercise for the healthy adult are three sessions of aerobic exercise for a minimum of 20 minutes every week. Aerobic exercise is any activity that raises the heartbeat above normal resting rate. There are three kinds of fitness: strength, stamina and suppleness. Activities to improve strength include working out at the gym; stamina – walking, running, swimming; and suppleness – yoga and Pilates. No matter what occupation, a good fitness regime incorporates elements from each group, done on a regular basis.

AIR

Bodies need food, air and water! We all know this, but it is easy to take for granted too. The brain needs a regular supply of oxygen and nutrients in order to function properly – in fact the brain consumes more oxygen than any other organ in the body. Oxygen is supplied in the air we breathe, and breathing is affected by posture and heart rate. If the rib cage is compressed, which happens if the body is slumped over, the lungs cannot take in as much oxygen as when the body is upright. Heart rate increases with activity, so a sedentary occupation requires less from the heart, and therefore lungs. But breathing is one of the few bodily activities that we can consciously control, and thus increase the amount of oxygen taken into the body. Incidentally, breathing consciously also affects the autonomic nervous system, and help lower stress levels.

FOOD

What you eat, how often, how much and when depends on individual belief, taste, sensitivity to certain foods, and metabolism, and despite the plethora of information available on diet and nutrition, each of us has to experiment to find what suits. Useful guidelines to remember in relation to working are that low blood sugar, or, for different reasons, a very full stomach, particularly of carbohydrates, can affect your concentration. Caffeine and sugar are nervous system stimulants and nicotine is a depressant; use of any of these before a session may impact on your ability to focus.

WATER

Dehydration also affects concentration. The recommendation to drink eight glasses of water a day may seem a lot, particularly if you're not used to it, but if you feel fuzzy or tired after a session it may be because your body is dehydrated. Have a glass of water and see if it makes a difference. Water in tea or coffee doesn't count, but does if drunk in herb tea. One practitioner I know drinks a glass between each client as a sort of cleansing ritual, as well as an automatic reminder to keep her water intake up.

Basic self care: taking stock exercise

Take some time to reflect on how you look after your body. Take a sheet of paper and divide it into three columns. Head the first one 'What I do now', the next one 'If I really loved myself I would…' and the last one 'One thing I will do in the next week'. Write down your answers in each of the following areas, and make a promise to yourself to change one small thing.

1. Exercise
   What sort and how often? Do you do a range of exercise, including cardiovascular strength and suppleness?

2. Diet
   Do you eat a balanced diet? Be honest! Do you eat regularly and, most importantly, enjoy it?

3. Water
   Is your intake enough to keep you from getting dehydrated? Do you feel thirsty during the day?

4. Air
   Like all living beings we need fresh air. Oxygen is essential for healthy cell metabolism. Do you spend time in fresh air each day? If you live in a city, are there times when you get out into green spaces, to replenish your oxygen supply?

5. Sleep
   Do you wake up refreshed? Are you getting the right amount of sleep for your needs? Do you have trouble getting to sleep or waking up?

6. Relaxation
   How do you relax? And how do you play? What sort of down time do you have and how often?

Self care of the mind

MENTAL EXERCISE

Taking care of your mind seems like a strange idea – aerobics or yoga for the mind? Well, yes, actually. The different aspects of our mind – and I'm not embarking on any discussion here about the nature, location or existence, even, of mind or of its relation to the body, I'm talking about mind in its common-sense form, the thing that does our thinking and which we assume is located in our head and is definitely something to do with the brain – this mind does need exercise and it does need to relax. We need to take care of our minds just as much as our bodies and include activities that promote both stretching and relaxation. A few years back I did a module of an MSc course which involved reading several research papers each week for discussion and writing a couple of essays. It was difficult at first but I soon found myself enjoying the intellectual challenge, and I began to think of my mind as a muscle. Doing this course was the equivalent of taking my rational mind to the gym regularly, as a result of which it got big and strong, and I knew that when I stopped, that aspect would atrophy again. For this reason, people who have retired are encouraged to do crosswords daily to keep their minds active. Unused neural circuits do eventually die, so it is a matter of use it or lose it. The rational mind needs exercising to keep in shape for the job, and the same is true of the intuitive mind. For many of us, this particular mind muscle is woefully underdeveloped, because we were never taught how to use it in school. The one instruction that all my subsequent teachers have given about using intuition is 'Just trust it!' Jessica Macbeth, author of *Moon Over Water* (2002) used to tell funny stories about trusting her intuition, like the time she found herself instructing a woman who'd come to consult her about her sick cat to go home and feed it spinach. Even as she said it her rational mind was saying 'Spinach? Cats don't eat spinach. Don't be ridiculous.' But the cat recovered, and, who knows, maybe the spinach had something to do with it.

MENTAL RELAXATION

The mind also needs to relax. A muscle that is continuously worked runs out of oxygen, builds up lactic acid, gets sore and is susceptible to injury. Minds also like to relax. They appreciate being unhooked from day-to-day thinking and allowed to float free and empty, like a blue morning sky, waiting for thoughts to arise. This form of attention is the basis of many meditation practices. Stilling the monkey mind, as it is sometimes called, the mind that chatters endlessly about this and that, bringing snippets of yesterday's conversation, concerns about coming events, memories triggered by something in the visual field, is not only a form of mental relaxation, it provides space for the other kinds of thought to arise, the intuitive ones, the sudden insights. To demonstrate how monkey mind works, catch yourself thinking about something and then backtrack your thought process. You may be surprised at its randomness. One neuron fires and triggers a set of responses in a chain of other neurons in the brain until the thought you end up with is far removed from the thought you started with. Learning to meditate is a way to halt these random mental processes, and is good discipline for the mind, whether as a tool to use in sessions or as a resource, a way of switching off.

SLEEP

The mind also needs good quality and sufficient sleep. Sleep deprivation studies show that lack of sleep affects the frontal cortex of the brain, and memory, speech production and problem solving become impaired. The ability to metabolise glucose drops, along with energy levels, and the sleep-deprived person feels tired, irritable and low. Although the number of hours needed a night differs for different people, on average eight to nine hours is required. This drops with age. People over 65 need only six to eight hours. Sleep hygiene recommendations to increase your chances for a good night's rest are to rest according to a schedule so that your body clock establishes a regular rhythm, eat your last meal several hours before bedtime, so that your body isn't busy digesting the food, and don't drink at bedtime, so a full bladder doesn't wake you up later.

Exercise to explore how you care for your mind

1. Write a list of all the ways in which you exercise or stretch your rational mind. This might include professional duties, like reading research reports, writing a teaching plan, devising aims and objectives for a course of treatment with a client book and recreational ones, like doing crosswords.

2. Write a list of all the ways you exercise your intuitive mind. This might include daydreaming, visualisation, and creative endeavours like writing a play, painting, making a garden.

3. Write a list of all the ways you relax your mind. This doesn't mean watching television! The brain is bombarded with visual and auditory signals from the screen, which are anything but restful. How do you switch off? If you really loved yourself, how would you look after your mind better? Think of one thing you could begin to do this very week.

Resources

What is a resource? Put simply, it's something that makes you feel better. Our self-care routines may be resources, but often they are things we do out of habit, paying little attention to what we are doing or how it makes us feel. Sometimes it depends on our intention. For example, a bath can be a rushed affair with the sole purpose of getting clean or it can be time out for yourself, an oasis of calm, when you turn the phones off and fill the bath with oils and surround it with candles. For some people a good dinner will be a resource, something that gives great pleasure, an event to be savoured in memory. For others, dinner might be a necessary daily ritual. A resource is something you can rely on, draw on or utilise to maintain or improve your physical, mental, emotional or spiritual well being. Different things work for different people. A resource can be real in the material world, a tangible object like a pebble kept in a pocket to hold in times of stress, a garden you visited for its tranquility, or a particular t-shirt that makes you feel good when you wear it. A resource can be a physical activity: running, dancing, doing yoga, lying on the earth, climbing mountains, walking, playing team sports, gardening or swimming. People can be resources; a teacher or supervisor, a good friend, your mum. Sometimes a resource might be an activity that you can lose yourself in, forgetting all other concerns, something so absorbing that you feel refreshed afterwards. Meditation is a good example, but for some people this could be making a model airplane, writing a poem, listening to music, and watching the grass grow. And a resource can be, very simply, a thought. This particular type of resource doesn't require special equipment, or travel to a particular place; it's one that can be used right now, wherever you are and whatever you're doing.

SPECIAL RESOURCES: STRAWBERRIES

Our thoughts affect our bodies. In Winnie the Pooh, Eeyore the donkey is depressed; he thinks gloomy, pessimistic thoughts. Pooh, on the other hand, with his mind on honey and snack time, is a happy little optimist. Positive thinking releases internal feel-good chemicals. This doesn't mean ignoring painful realities to live in cloud cuckoo land. Our professional selves encounter pain, distress, all sorts of physical suffering, dying and death, and each of us has to find our own way to be comfortable with these things and compassionate to those who suffer and to ourselves as witnesses. We also have a responsibility to ourselves to think positive. An accumulation of stress chemicals in the system leads to disease over time, as we all know. Why release more when you could choose to do otherwise? As William Bloom (2001), one of Britain's leading holistic teachers, says: 'The pressures of daily human existence create tension and block the flow of endorphins and benevolent vitality... (p.60) "Loving yourself", then, is not some touchy feely irrelevance. It is a practical method of inducing relaxation and health' (p.99).

In his book *The Endorphin Effect* he calls resources strawberries, which are 'anything or any thought that brings you pleasure, makes you smile, opens your heart and makes you feel good about life' (p.74). An inner strawberry, a thought or memory, has a similar effect on the body as a real bright red juicy strawberry.

✍ **Inner strawberry exercise**

1. Remember the last time you felt really good. Maybe last week at dinner with friends, or when your team won a match, when you got better exam results than you'd expected, or after a day sunbathing or last time a child made you laugh.

2. Sit comfortably and relax your body. Now bring your chosen memory to mind. Visualise it as fully as you can, including sounds, scents, textures and feel, as well as the visual aspect.

3. Notice sensations in your body. Notice how you feel.

SPECIAL RESOURCES: ANCHORS

Babette Rothschild, international teacher of somatic trauma therapy, uses a similar concept with people who have been traumatised. She relates use of resources to autonomic nervous system activity. She uses the word 'anchor' for thoughts about a person, animal, activity, or place that make a person feel good. People who have been traumatised live in a constant state of hyperarousal, with their nervous systems jammed on alert and unable to switch off. Talking about the trauma increases, rather than releases, the feelings associated with the initial events. We may all have had a taste of this after major disasters like 9/11, or the London train bombings, when many people found themselves becoming overwhelmed by the repetition of images and constant replaying of the events by the media, and affected as if they had actually been present. Thinking about a resource releases the feel-good chemicals which temporarily switch off a hyperarousal state in the body, thus anchoring the traumatised person in the here and now, and moving her away from overwhelming feelings. An anchor is a thought which cuts through an anxiety cycle, bringing the person back to earth. An anchor is a grounding thought.

The other day I used an anchor activity without meaning to. I was listening to Roger, a psychotherapy client, a man who was brought up in four different foster homes and who gets very anxious about breaks in his therapy because they remind him of the many times he lost his 'family'. It's as if the small boy in him still doesn't trust that I won't send him packing to another 'mum' when I go on holiday. He was talking very fast about all sorts of things that were making him feel scared, including our forthcoming holiday, when I remembered that he'd been due to collect new kittens that weekend. I interrupted him to ask if they'd arrived. He affirmed that they had and began to talk about them, his face softening into a smile, his speech slowing, his body opening out. It was clear that the thought of the kittens was acting as an internal anchor, breaking through his anxiety.

✍ Exercise to find your own resources

It doesn't matter what you call your own resources – strawberries, anchors or something else – but it is important that you can identify them, the things in your life that give you pleasure, make you feel good about being here, and that improve your health by changing your internal chemistry.

Take some time to reflect on this, and make lists, using the following headings:

- objects
- people
- activities
- places
- other.

Now choose the 'best' one, whatever that is for you, close your eyes and imagine it, as fully as you can. Observe your internal response. How do you know that this makes you feel good? What happens in your body? What sensations are you aware of? There will be some kind of change as different chemicals and nerve paths get triggered by the thought, but how you experience this is yours alone. Some people feel warmth in their tummy, others tingling or expansion around the heart area, and others still a glow permeating the whole body. What's your feel-good experience?

How could you bring more of this into your life?

Professional self care

In the previous section we looked at basic self care and resources. We need to keep ourselves healthy and balanced to do our work. In fact, most professional codes of conduct state that the therapist has a responsibility to look after herself to ensure that she is fit to work. Here are two examples.

The Massage Training Institute:
Practitioners must ensure they are competent to give massage in the best interests of the client. If this is not possible, through ill health – mentally or physically – the practitioner should refrain from practising.

The Craniosacral Therapy Association UK:
We take care of our own health and recognise that this is our responsibility, both for our own sake and that of our clients.

What does your professional self look like?

We all have many aspects to our self, which come out in different situations. We are all someone's child and in the presence of a parent can find ourselves reverting to behaviours that we thought we had long grown out of. How we are with a lover, the assistant in the supermarket and a prospective employer varies, sometimes in obvious ways, sometimes subtly. The same is true for our professional selves. Do you know the face you put on for clients? These two exercises help you to contact the part of yourself that is a professional, and to explore how you see yourself, possibly without knowing it, as a health-care practitioner (therapist, healer, practitioner or whatever term applies).

Exercise to discover your professional self – method one

Sit quietly and bring your awareness into your breathing and into your body. Allow your mind to quieten. When you are ready imagine that you are sitting in a little film studio, facing a blank white screen. There's no one else present. As you watch the screen an image begins to appear. This is you as a therapist (practitioner, health-care professional). The image might jump onto the screen, or it might emerge slowly. The image may be still or moving. Don't judge, just observe it. Notice your reactions to the image. When you are ready, bring your attention back to the room and write down what you noticed.

Exercise to discover your professional self – method two

This may be easier if you find visualisation hard. Sit quietly and bring your awareness into your breathing and into your body. Allow your mind to quieten. Imagine you are sitting in your workspace, resting between clients, having a cup of tea and perhaps reading the paper or listening to some music. You have an hour before the next client. Or so you believe. The bell/phone rings and your next person is waiting. As you shift from your quiet private world into work mode, observe the changes that take place. How does your body change? Your facial expression? What happens to your thought processes? Are there any energetic shifts? When you have finished observing, bring your attention back to the room and write down what you noticed.

You may like to use the following questions to help you understand what you noticed:

1. Was there anything that surprised you?
2. What did the image in method one mean to you? Did you like it? If not, why?
3. Were the changes in method two comfortable?
4. Is there anything you want to change after doing these exercises?

Here are two examples from colleagues who tried the exercises. David visualised his practitioner self on a screen: he saw himself sitting at a table with a cup of tea, talking to someone, no massage table in sight. He was pleased with the image, understanding it to be an affirmation of his belief that the most important aspect of his work as a practitioner was to be with someone, nothing more, and nothing less. In the second exercise, Sue described her energy as flowing up and forward from a diffuse resting in her whole body to settle in her face and the front of her chest area, a bit like a shield. She realised it was a form of protection, but that it left her lower body exposed.

Self care of your professional body

How do you use your body during your work? If your therapy is one that involves a lot of sitting, do the chairs or stools you use support your back properly? If your work is mainly sedentary, are you making sure you move or stretch between sessions and do some cardiovascular exercise regularly? If your body is a tool for the treatment, are you using it in a way that avoids strain, repetitive injuries or imbalance? If the good habits you learned at the beginning of your training are slipping, or you find yourself with aches and pains at the end of the day, think about finding alternative ways of doing techniques that are problematic, or ask a colleague to observe you and recommend changes of body use, or compensating exercises.

And how many of us receive the therapy we practise ourselves on a regular basis? It's important to keep in mind the experience of being a client, to know what it feels like to be on the receiving end in the therapeutic relationship. It's also important to receive some kind of therapy for ourselves to prevent an unacknowledged resentment from building up.

Professional resources

These are the things or people that make you feel good about yourself as a practitioner, that give you confidence, remind you of your value, fire up your passion for the work and generally support you. Different resources are needed at different times. The practitioner who has just qualified and is beginning her practice needs encouragement and support from others who are further down the road and have already dealt with the sorts of problems she's encountering. The practitioner who's been in business for many years has needs to do with maintaining excitement and curiosity in the work, preventing burn out, learning new therapies, or working with different client groups. All of us need support and help when things get tough, or we are unsure of ourselves.

✍ **Exercise to explore your professional resources**

  1. Think about and make a list of all the resources that support you in your work as a complementary therapist. Use the following headings:

       ° colleagues

       ° websites

- ◦ journals, books
- ◦ networking
- ◦ supervision
- ◦ continuing professional development (CPD) – courses, conferences, workshops
- ◦ other.

2. Go through the list again, noting how often you use each resource. Once a month when your professional journal comes through the door? Once in a blue moon when you have coffee with a colleague?

3. Think of one thing you could do to improve your professional resources.

Supervision

This is a resource that is, I think, underrated and consequently underused by complementary therapists. The word itself is a bit unattractive, with its connotations of control, management and regulation. There are alternatives that suggest a friendlier relationship: mentoring, support, and consultancy. But supervision is the term currently in use, so I'll stick with it here.

In many professions supervision is mandatory. The British Association of Counselling and Psychotherapy requires its members to be in regular and ongoing supervision. Craniosacral therapists are required to have supervision throughout their first year after qualification. Good supervision instils genuine confidence, enables a person to identify weaknesses and find ways to overcome or compensate for them and renews flagging enthusiasm. A good supervisor is a resource, a shoulder to cry on, a listening ear, and provides time out to be still and listen to your inner voice.

There are several methods of supervision. Peer supervision refers to two or more colleagues meeting to talk about work. This requires some discipline to ensure that the time isn't taken up drinking tea and gossiping. Ground rules have to be established about how much time each person gets to talk, or agreement about a topic for discussion and so on. The advantages of peer supervision are that it is free, and talking to people in the same situation can feel more supportive and equal. On the other hand, the advice, resources and degree of support is more limited than that available from a longer standing colleague. Then there is the supervision that is a formal, paid arrangement with someone who is more experienced, and who may have a qualification or done some training in supervision. In this relationship, the supervisor has a degree of responsibility for the practitioner and her work. Both peer and formal supervision can be one to one, or in a group. The former provides individual time and attention and the latter the opportunity of learning from others in the group.

What are the functions of supervision? Support is one of the main aspects, both practical and emotional. The new practitioner, having left the comfort and security of the training group, may find setting up a practice or finding clients or work a bit of a struggle. A supervisor may be able to give useful suggestions about marketing, websites and publicity, or recommend clinics or centres that may rent space. He or she can help with the little problems that everyone encounters at the beginning. Here are some examples. Paul was dyslexic and, despite his specially designed computer programs, always took his publicity material to his supervisor to check. Shelley had rented space in a health centre, and when a number of clients cancelled, she found herself out of pocket. She needed to work out a cancellation policy that suited her, and a way to communicate this to clients. Her supervisor helped her by doing role-plays until Shelley found the way to communicate which was professional, and the right balance of assertive and friendly.

If you see the same supervisor over time, he or she develops an overview of your work and, from this perspective, can provide advice about your ongoing professional development. He or she could point you in the direction of books, articles or postgraduate workshops in your line of interest, or help you liaise with other practitioners if you are working in a specialist field, or suggest that you investigate other complementary therapies to stimulate new learning.

Emotional support is also important. The life of a complementary therapist can be lonely. Some of us work in centres where we can chat to others in our breaks and a few may be part of a care team and take part in regular case meetings, but many of us work in isolation. The stories our clients tell us are confidential, and it wouldn't be right – or professional – to go home and repeat what we hear to our nearest and dearest. But sometimes we can only bear to witness so much of others' pain and suffering without getting overwhelmed. Whatever other resources we may have, a good supervisor is invaluable at this point. Like the client/practitioner relationship, everything that gets spoken in the supervisee/supervisor relationship is also confidential. Just sharing with another person, especially one who may have had similar experiences, mitigates the isolation and provides a space to unburden. This applies particularly to people working with certain client groups. People in recovery from substance abuse, those with a terminal illness and the recently bereaved can trigger issues for all of us.

Good supervision sometimes encompasses both emotional and practical support. Here's an example. John was a single parent and newly qualified homeopath. We spent a lot of time in his supervision sessions discussing the pros and cons of different clinics where he could work and how the times would fit in with his child-care arrangements, but I suspected that underlying his practical concerns was his lack of confidence, so I'd ask him to shut his eyes and imagine himself in each venue then check in with his body to see how comfortable he felt there. Sure enough, the clinics that he chose to work in were those that supported rather than demanded too much of him.

Supervision can be educational. Kelly, one of my supervisees, was contacted by a young woman with a severe scoliosis supported by a metal rod next to the spine. Several beauty therapy salons in central London had refused to massage her. Kelly was very anxious that she'd do something to harm her. We discussed the things she needed to ask in the case history, including permission to liaise with the woman's doctor. Then we took it in turn to imagine ourselves into the client's body and, lying on the couch, experimented with cushions and pillows to see what sort of support she might need.

Sometimes supervision can help with ethical matters. Fran, a young supervisee, was a body psychotherapist, using massage to facilitate emotional release. She arrived one day highly agitated, crying, 'I've really blown it this time! I've broken all the rules!' When she calmed down I learned about her session with Bill, an ongoing client, the previous day. Bill was in his sixties and had mild cerebral palsy. During the massage he'd got an erection and had asked Fran to look at it. Intuitively, she'd felt this was the right thing to do. Just for a moment she uncovered his penis then replaced the towel. But after he left she panicked and had fantasies about being struck off her register. I too wondered about the ethics of her behaviour. As we talked, Bill's story and the possible reason behind his request emerged. He was ashamed of his twisted body and part of his reason for working with Fran was to have his body witnessed compassionately. He had never had a sexual relationship with a woman. Maybe he just wanted his sexuality to be witnessed as well? Fran certainly hadn't felt abused or taken advantage of by his request. We decided that she should talk with Bill about the incident and, if necessary, state clearly what was acceptable (witnessing) and what wasn't (touching, or anything further). She needed to be clear in herself that she had a professional and not a sexual relationship with Bill. We role-played the best ways for her to communicate this to him.

How to find a supervisor? If your issues are practical or related to your therapeutic skills, contact your professional organisation. If you need emotional support, or have difficulties within the therapeutic relationship, you could contact the British Association of Counselling and Psychotherapy (BACP) for a list of supervisors in your area. A competent supervisor wouldn't need to know too much about the therapy you practise to help you in these areas.

Burn out

When a practitioner reaches this stage it indicates that she hasn't been taking care or using her resources, and needs to stop. Hypocrates didn't say 'physician, heal thyself' for nothing. We are no use to our clients if we are burnt out.

The warning signs to watch out for include:

- Exhaustion, tiredness, forgetfulness, feeling run down.

- Difficulty sleeping. Thoughts going round and round all night long.

- Feeling on edge much of the time, easily irritated or weepy, or having emotional outbursts.

- Feeling bored and cynical about work.

- Appetite and weight changes, either gain or loss.

- Increased illnesses like colds and stomach upsets.

- Having no patience with clients who complain about their lot.

If you find yourself exhibiting any of these signs, do something about it. Heroism has no place in the complementary therapy treatment room. Take a break, rest, reduce your client load, go swimming, walking, for a massage – use your resources and get your energy back.

Self care and resources for the therapeutic relationship

I'm going to suggest another aspect of self care, one we need in order to work with the therapeutic relationship. These are skills that psychotherapists and counsellors learn as part of their training which help them to use their own thoughts, feelings and messages from the body to understand what might be going on for another person. The more self awareness a therapist, of any kind, possesses, the easier it is for her to understand and use all the information that arises in the presence of a client. We aren't psychotherapists, we don't work with our clients' emotional and psychological processes (I know some homeopaths might disagree with me here) but we can use these techniques to work with our own internal processes.

Let's begin by acknowledging the body as a therapeutic tool, not merely the vehicle that houses the complementary therapist's mind, but very much part of the process when it comes to a treatment session. Your body is the origin of the feelings, hunches, empathetic responses and emotional (gut) reactions to what happens between you and the patient, and your mind is the aspect that makes sense of all this material. I know that the more I am able to stay connected to my own body, to monitor ongoing impulses from my gut, heart, breathing and muscular tension, the better I am able to 'read' the situation and, importantly, to recognise if my somatic reactions are a result of my own process being triggered or are something I am 'picking up' from the other person. Sometimes these somatic sensations stay with me after a session, like memories that I can't put on one side.

How to be your own inner therapist

In order to understand what is going on in the relationships you have with your clients some psychological theory is helpful, knowledge of ethics and legalities provide an essential framework but the main tool you have is yourself and your felt lived experience in the treatment room, and the ability to reflect on your experience. Contemplation of your thoughts, attitudes, beliefs and prejudices and the willingness to change them isn't just help about acquiring more tricks for your therapeutic tool box; it also helps you recognise who you are as a human being. It helps to cultivate the following:

1. Being grounded and centred. In this state nothing knocks you off balance. Having a firm inner core, a place where you stand, not rigidly but with flexibility and lightness.

2. Mindfulness. The ability to be 100 per cent present with what really is, without judging it.

3. Awareness of somatic sensation. Many of us live predominantly in our heads even though we work with other people's bodies. Knowing what our body is feeling, being able to tune inwardly at the same time as our attention is focused outwards, offers invaluable information about what is going on, especially how we feel about it.

4. Focusing. This is a form of self reflection arising from somatic sensation.

The importance of grounding

Grounding means being connected to the earth in such a way that nothing can blow you over, undermine you, overwhelm you and cause you to wobble. Think of a large old oak tree in the middle of a field in midsummer. Strong winds, gales even, disturb the leaves, snap off dead branches, maybe bend the trunk, but cannot knock the tree over. Its roots hold firm in the earth. When we are grounded we can listen to all kinds of material without getting lost or over-whelmed. We are able to walk around inside another's world, while never losing a sense of our self and our own experience as separate. We need to be firmly rooted but also flexible. Too rigid and we snap; not enough base and we get blown away.

How do you know when you are grounded? You may already have regular grounding exercises that you do at the beginning of the day or before each client. Grounding exercises vary from elaborate visualisations to feeling the soles of the feet in contact with the floor. Try this one to test the effectiveness of your grounding.

Grounding exercise

Stand and spend as long as it takes to do your own grounding exercise. Then be aware how your body feels. Let your attention move around, noticing sensations in your legs, trunk, head and shoulders and arms. What's your breathing like? Notice your emotional state. What word would you use to describe your emotional state right now? Notice your energy. Where is your energy centred in your body right now?

Then I'd like you to imagine you're running though a crowded station to catch a train. You've got two heavy bags, banging against your legs. The train leaves in three minutes and you can't find the platform. People are bumping into you and standing in your way. It's very important that you don't miss this train. Bring your attention back to your body and notice how it feels now. Notice sensations in your legs, trunk, head and shoulders and arms. What's your breathing like? Notice your emotional state. What word would you use to describe your emotional state right now? Notice your energy. Where is your energy centred in your body right now?

The importance of centering

Not quite the same as grounding, which is about our relationship to the earth, being centred refers to the ability to sit in the core of yourself, to experience the centre of your being as a physical reality. For some people this might be their belly, for some the heart centre, for others the third eye, in the middle of the forehead.

Exercise to ground and centre
(With thanks to Jessica Macbeth)

Sit comfortably – cross-legged or in a straight back chair with both feet flat on the floor, in a quiet room, with your spine erect. Rest your hands in your lap. Notice sounds around you. Bring your attention to your body and, if there's anything you can do to make yourself more comfortable, do it now. Become aware of your breathing – you don't have to change it, your body knows how to breathe. Just watch it. Then bring your attention to the base of your spine, in between your sitting bones and let it rest there for a moment. You might feel tingling or warmth or you might not, it doesn't matter. Now imagine a line, or a cord, or a thread, extending out from that place down into the earth, directly into the floor if you are cross-legged, or down through your legs and out of the soles of your feet if sitting. Imagine this line descending through floors, foundations of the building into the earth and like the roots of a tree, moving down, spreading out and anchoring you firmly. Rest with this sensation for a moment. Now bring your attention back up through the roots, back up the line into your body. Imagine the line continuing upwards through the very centre of your body, through your belly, diaphragm, chest, neck into your head. Up it goes to the crown of your head, then upwards still, into the air above you. Imagine an energy source somewhere above your head; you might like to call it heaven, or universal energy, or god, or cosmic love, it really doesn't matter. Just imagine your line reaching up to this source and as you do so, you may feel the back of your neck elongating and your head lifting. Be aware of the line connecting you to the earth and the heavens, and let yourself experience this connection for a few moments. Now let your attention move up and down the line within your physical body until you find a spot that feels like your centre, the core of your being. There isn't a right or wrong about this, there's just your centre, the place you identify as home in your body. When you have found it, rest there for a few moments. Now open your eyes very slowly, keeping an awareness of your centre and your connection to heaven and earth and look at the world from this place. How does it feel?

Mindfulness

For in the dew of little things the heart finds its morning and is refreshed.
(Kahlil Gibran, *The Prophet*, p.70)

Mindfulness is being fully conscious in the present moment, and aware of the world around and within you. Mindfulness is paying attention to all your senses: to what you can see, hear, smell, touch, taste, and to the sense of movement in your body. Mindfulness is being here and now without the distractions of thoughts and memories. Mindfulness is a practice that helps us to become still, and to focus. It helps us to feel fully alive in the moment.

We live in a visually dominated world. Once upon a time we relied on our sense of smell and taste for our survival: the smell of other creatures, friendly or dangerous, the taste of good or bad food. These days survival depends on being able to see the traffic; much of information about the distant world is received visually, on television, websites and in newspapers. We also rely less on our sense of hearing. Mindfulness helps us reconnect to those senses that have been relegated to second place. It is a form of meditation, but, unlike forms of meditation that focus on emptying the mind, or on stilling the activity by concentrating on a single entity – a mantra, or the breath – mindfulness focuses on the external world as perceived through our senses.

Like all forms of meditation, mindfulness seems very hard initially. The mind wanders, the habitual thought processes re-establish, and distractions are suddenly everywhere. There's a temptation to give up, or to get irritated with yourself. Instead, gently bring the mind back to the present. Just notice where you are at the moment: your surroundings, who you are with, what you can hear, what you can feel in contact with your body. Know that this moment is unique: you have never been in this place in this way before, and never will be again.

Mindfulness is relevant to complementary therapists because it fosters the ability to be present in the moment with our client, without judgement. Mindfulness is unconditional – we notice what is, without prejudice. For many of us, the experience of receiving another's total unconditional attention and presence is rare – if we can transmit even a little of this to the people we work with through being mindful, we give them a true gift.

Mindfulness exercises

1. Stand up and feel the contact of your bare feet on the ground. Lift your toes, stretch them out, place them down, and feel the contact again. Slowly begin to walk. Be aware of the sensations of pressure on the soles changing as your weight shifts from heel to toes. Notice if there are places where you begin to wobble. Walk around the room, staying mindful of your feet contacting the ground.

2. Choose any object or surface – the table, the door, a cup, a plant, it doesn't matter. Sit comfortably, and look at your chosen object. Really look. Let your eyes notice colours, textures, shapes, surfaces. Become aware of things you wouldn't normally notice. Spend a few minutes just looking.

3. Choose a piece of music to play. Lie down, close your eyes and just listen. Give yourself permission to not think about anything. Just follow the sounds and rhythms.

4. Take an everyday activity, like cleaning your teeth. Stay mindful of what you are doing as you do it. Notice each tiny portion of the activity – the feel of your arm as you reach for the toothbrush, the smoothness of the toothbrush, the sound of the tap water, the smell of the toothpaste, and so on.

5. When you next eat something, take time to feel the texture as you bite, the movement of your jaws as you chew, the taste in your mouth, the feel as you swallow. Take time, too, to chew really well. How often do you really notice what you are eating?

Somatic awareness

The mindfulness exercises remind us that our bodies receive input from the external world through many channels. And they also have sense receptors in every inch of skin, in our guts, muscles and joints, blood vessels and all our organs. Our brains receive information from all these little nerves equally, but we pay far more attention to the input from the sense organs in our head than we do to the others. Once upon a time, when we lived simpler lives, without the sheer volume of visual and auditory stimuli that bombard us today, we probably paid far more attention to the input from the rest of our bodies. Imagine a world where the only stimuli from the environment are the light changing throughout the day, the feel of rain, and the noise of the wind. In such a world it would be so much easier to focus on our own inner sensations, to be conscious of the interface between inner and outer. Today we hardly ever experience complete silence or darkness. There are continual demands on our senses, particularly those located in our heads, to deal with the never ending procession of sights, sounds, smells, and tastes, and our ability to focus on our inner world has atrophied. Many of us find it difficult to live fully in our bodies. It takes time, patience and trust to come back into relationship with our bodies.

There are also people who are too scared to come back into relationship with their bodies, for fear of what they might find there. And people who hate or are disgusted by their bodies to such an extent that the only thing they want to do is disown them. And people who not only 'live in their heads' but who can leave their bodies altogether when things get too difficult. People who have been traumatised – and the list of events that can be traumatic includes physical neglect as well as mental, emotional and physical abuse; invasive medical treatments; living with a life threatening or terminal illness; being in an accident or fire; torture; or witnessing many of these – may find the focusing process overwhelming and may need to work with someone trained in shock and trauma.

There's an exercise that I often do at the beginning of a treatment, with a new client, partly because the focus takes him out of his head, which in itself is often relaxing (but not for everyone: some people live in their heads because the body is a terrifying place, full of unknown sensations and feelings, and for them, a body-focusing exercise induces agitation, not calm) but also to see how in touch he is with his body. Not surprisingly, many people can't sense all their body, or can't get their attention below their neck. This includes practitioners who work with other people's bodies. When I was first in practice, I could only sense my body as far as my collarbones. It took a long time before I really inhabited my whole being.

✍ **Body sensation exercise**
Lie comfortably on your back. Notice the contact that the back of your head makes with the couch (pillow, floor). Roll your head slightly side to side if you can't feel anything. Let your attention move round your head, noticing how your scalp feels, the little muscles round your eyes and mouth, on your forehead. Notice your jaw and throat. Don't judge, just observe. Now let your attention move down into your throat and neck and see what's going on there. Then down into your chest and across your shoulders. Move your attention into your left arm, from the shoulder down through your elbow to your left wrist and hand. Then do the same with your right arm. Bring your attention into your ribcage. Notice how your body moves as you breathe. You don't have to change anything – your body knows how to breathe. Let your attention fall into your back – your shoulder blades, spine, lower back, the contact they make with the couch. Bring your attention to your belly. Be aware of any sensations in this part of your body. Move down to your pelvic area, your hips, your buttocks and genitals. Not judging, just noticing. Move down to your thighs, knees, calves and feet. Then get a sense of your whole body, as it is right now.

The following questions may give you some interesting information about your body. Was there anything that drew your attention strongly while you did the exercise? Were there places that you found hard to focus on, or that didn't seem to be present, or where you found your mind wandering? Did you notice any difference between your left and right side? Where would you say you live in your body?

And then there's the question of making sense of the sensations. Some of us are so out of touch that we haven't learned how to listen to our bodies. Kelly was a young woman who had survived a very chaotic, insecure and abusive childhood by dissociating from her body, like so many children in that situation. She described looking down on what was happening, like a fly on the wall. Kelly had been so out of touch with her body that she hadn't learned to recognise such common signals as hunger, a full bladder or tiredness. If we are to stay grounded, connected to the earth, and centred in our own bodies, we need to be familiar with our own sensation repertoire. Sometimes I give people the following exercise, to help connect to the vocabulary about sensations.

✍ **Words for sensations exercise**
Write down as many words as you can think of to describe felt sensations in the body:

  ○ in muscles, e.g. sore
  ○ in your chest, e.g. tight
  ○ in your tummy, e.g. full

- in your feet, e.g. tired
- in your face, e.g. hot
- in your head, e.g. buzzy
- any other words.

Focusing

Eugene Gendlin (1978), one of the founders of neuro-linguistic programming, developed a form of self reflection called focusing, which utilises body sensations, bringing them into awareness and connecting them with emotion, memory or meaning.

The process of bringing felt bodily sensations into conscious awareness is a skill that, like any skill, becomes easier with practice. Understanding of a felt sensation can happen at any point during the process. The message from the body may be urgent and immediate. If you have been 'in your head' all morning, working on the computer perhaps, then just sitting quiet and focusing may bring to awareness the sensation of full bladder and dry throat. No points for working out the message!

Sometimes the message may come in a flash. For example, Sara was focusing on a sensation of tightness and soreness around her breastbone, which spread to a constriction in her throat, when a sudden memory of her mother sprang into her mind, and the tears came. When she had finished crying, she remembered that it was the anniversary of her mother's death.

And sometimes the meaning takes a while to emerge. Gerry had a sore elbow joint that didn't seem to be postural or work related and massage gave temporary relief. Focusing on the sensation produced lurching feelings in his stomach and a sensation of shock, which didn't make any sense. Several days later he was walking past a pub and remembered drinking there the previous month; then he also remembered that when he left, slightly the worse for wear, he'd slipped over and had fallen onto his elbow. Bringing this event back into consciousness, and acknowledging the shock, helped his elbow to heal.

✍ Focusing exercise

1. Sit comfortably in a quiet place and shut your eyes. Bring your awareness to sensations from the world around you; notice what you can hear, smell, and feel on the skin of your face. Notice sensations at the interface of your body with its surroundings; the pressure of your buttocks and thighs on the chair/floor, the feel of your arms against your body, the feel of fabrics against your skin. Bring your awareness into your body; notice your breath, and the movements of your body as you breathe. Try not to judge any of it; be an impartial witness.

2. Allow your awareness to float freely within your body and wait for something to attract your attention. A particularly strong or insistent sensation, perhaps, or an ache, or a discomfort, or an energetic charge. Bring all your awareness to rest in that part of your body, in that sensation. (An alternative way to begin, if the above seems too vague, or you find yourself drifting off, is to start by bringing your awareness to the top of your head and noticing any sensations in your scalp and skull. Bring your attention down into your face, the little muscles around your eyes, nose and mouth and the place where your jaw hinges. Continue right down to your toes, scanning each part of your body in turn and then focus back on your whole body, and ask yourself which part seems to be demanding your attention.)

3. Focus on the sensation and wait. What words would you use to describe the sensation? Does it have a colour, shape, texture or movement? Be patient; stay with it and watch it with your inner eye; notice how it changes as you observe it.

4. Ask yourself how you feel about this sensation. Do you feel comfortable with it or uncomfortable? Is it pleasant or not? Can you identify any emotional feelings connected to it? See if a word comes to you to describe your emotional reaction to this sensation.

5. Does it remind you of anything? Have you experienced it before, and if so when? Allow any memories that may want to arise in connection with this sensation. Be an impartial witness, if you can; just watch the memories as if you are watching a slide show.

6. If you want to take the process a step further, imagine that you are sitting in a room facing a big blank screen. Let your awareness rest on the sensation again, then ask yourself if there is an image that represents this sensation. Watch the screen and wait to see what appears on it. Trust whatever comes, even if it appears to make no sense.

7. Bring your awareness back to your everyday surroundings. You may want to draw, write down or think about what you experienced.

Using focusing to clarify difficulties in a relationship

You can use this exercise with anyone you might be having problems with, particularly if there's something that's bothering you about the connection between you, and thinking about it doesn't help. If it's a problem with a client, then this exercise can shift things without you having to say anything to the person involved. If this sounds a bit magical, well, maybe it is.

You'll need a quiet place where you won't be disturbed, enough time – half an hour should be sufficient – and writing things, to make notes of your discoveries. This you could do between each part, or wait until you've finished. Remember that there isn't a right or wrong way to do this exercise, there is only your way. Trust your intuition, however silly the messages it gives you may seem.

Sit quietly, do whatever you do to ground and centre and let your thoughts settle. Now bring the other person to mind. You might remember the last time you saw him or her, or you might imagine them sitting or standing in front of you. Imagine them as fully as possible. Notice posture, body language, facial expression, and clothes. Is the person silent or talking? If talking what's the tone of voice? Spend some moments watching, listening, sensing their presence with you.

Now withdraw your attention from the other person and bring it back to yourself. Be aware of sensations in your body, particularly ones that seem to be associated with what's happening. Observe your muscles, particularly your jaw, shoulders, arms and back. Observe your heart and breathing rate. Observe sensations in your abdomen. Don't think too much about them, or try to understand them at this point. Notice the thoughts in your mind, letting them come and go, or go round in circles, or whatever they're doing.

Then ask yourself the following questions. Are these things that I'm experiencing familiar to me? Have I felt like this before, and if so, what does it remind me of? Wait for the answer to come, it might be immediate, or it might dawn on you slowly, or it might not. What you're experiencing might possibly not be anything to do with you.

When you're ready, take another look at the other person. Extend your attention out again. Has anything changed? It may not have, or you may find your perception of the other was altered. Then ask yourself if the feelings you've been experiencing are anything to do with the other persons. Is he or she trying to communicate anything? Wait and trust whatever comes to you.

The next question to ask yourself is whether there's anything that needs to be done now. This could mean having a dialogue right there and then with the other person in your imagination, it could mean making a note to talk to your supervisor about it, or it could mean something else altogether. Be patient and wait for the answer.

Finally, thank the other person for being with you and let them go. Imagine them walking away, or dissolving, or fading. Take a deep breath, come back psent and open your eyes.

3

Boundaries

There's an old custom, still observed in some country areas, called 'beating the bounds'. The whole village turns out on the specified day, and together they walk round the boundary of the village, reminding each other of their territory, of the edge between their land and that of their neighbour. Boundaries give shape to a particular space, and help to define its function. Boundaries usually refer to physical space. Near my house, Green Lanes marks the boundary between Islington and Hackney. My skin is the boundary between me and not me. Somewhere in the English Channel is the boundary between England and France. In Australia, a boundary rider is the person who maintains the fences on the perimeter of a sheep or cattle farm, to prevent the animals straying. A place that is 'out of bounds' is one that is forbidden territory.

Boundaries can also refer to the norms of behaviour, the unwritten rules of conduct that we absorb as children about how to be in the culture in which we're raised. In the English language there are phrases that point to this sense of boundaries between acceptable and non-acceptable behaviour. We talk about deviant behaviour as being 'beyond the pale'. We tell those who are provocative to 'stop pushing it' and we are careful not to 'overstep the mark'. The punishment of 'being sent to Coventry' excludes the unfortunate victim from the group. Cultural norms are so pervasive that we aren't aware of them until someone transgresses, or when we find ourselves in a country with very different assumptions about appropriate behaviour.

Boundaries are edges, and as well as defining what belongs inside the space and what stays outside, they also act as containers for the contents of the space in the same way, say, that the cell membrane allows in needed nutrients, keeps out unwanted chemicals, and contains the cytoplasm and nucleus of the cell. If the cell membrane is damaged, the contents leak out and the cell loses its integrity. The thicker and clearer the edges of any boundary, the safer are the contents. Soup won't last long in a sieve but does in a bowl, a pricked balloon soon deflates and the three little pigs were finally protected from the wicked wolf in a house of bricks and mortar.

What has all this got to do with relationships, and in particular, the therapeutic one? All relationships have certain things in common; they often take place in defined spaces, and there are assumptions on both sides about what sort of things take place between the two people. Consider the relationships you have with an elderly family member, your doctor, your brother (if you have one), your partner (if you have one) and a baby. Each has a distinctive quality that makes it different from the rest. Consider how you would greet each of those people. The choice of words, tone of voice and your physical behaviour would vary according to the person. You wouldn't shake hands with a serious 'good morning' with a baby, and neither would you gaze at your doctor, head on one side, and say, in a singsong voice, 'You're gorgeous, you are. Yes you are.'

The rules about appropriate interpersonal behaviour are seldom explained or taught once we're no longer children, except in certain unusual circumstances, such as attending a royal garden party, when it's important to know how to address royalty and whether to curtsy or not. Visiting a church, a mosque, a temple or a synagogue requires knowledge of the particular observances of that religion, in order to avoid offence.

By and large, complementary therapists aren't taught about the boundaries of the therapeutic relationship. Being 'professional' is often modelled on tutors' behaviour, or that of professionals we've been to as clients. If we apply the idea mentioned above (boundaries as outline, boundaries as defining contents and boundaries as a safe container) to the therapeutic relationship, then we are concerned with the following factors:

- Physical boundaries. The general environment, the treatment room, privacy, heating, lighting. The energy in the room.

- The contract, including time, money, confidentiality and the agreement between practitioner and client.

- Personal space. The practitioner and the client's physical, emotional and energetic boundaries.

Physical boundaries

The worst space I ever worked in was the back room of a small shop that had been roughly converted into an alternative health centre. The front room where the receptionist sat opened straight onto a busy main road, and the back room onto a parking lot. The walls badly needed painting, the carpet had seen better days and the toilet was grimy. I could hear the conversations of the receptionist word for word, despite the traffic rumble, and no doubt she could hear my discussions with clients too. I didn't stay there long. What's your worst treatment room memory?

If a room is to act as a secure container it must have doors which won't be opened during a treatment, windows with curtains or blinds to keep out the nosy world, if necessary, and phones that are switched off. Taking phone calls during a session allows the outside world in and conveys the message that you are not fully available to your client. The size of the room matters too. It must be big enough for the practical needs of your treatment, but not too big that it becomes impersonal or hard to heat. I hadn't realised how sensitive some people can be to the size of a room until I moved my practice from a small cosy room, where there was just enough space to move comfortably round the treatment couch, to a more spacious one. Even though I appreciated all the advantages I didn't like my new room. Several of my clients were also quite disturbed by the move. The room was just too big and we felt lost in it! I resolved the problem by pulling the couch over to the sitting area, thus delineating a smaller space within the room.

Secure boundaries are vital, but aesthetics matter too. You and your client would prefer to be in a room that looks and feels good. (Although it's surprising how little some people notice their environment. One woman who I'd seen for counselling for a few months suddenly said, noticing my massage table folded and leaning against the wall on the far side of the room, 'Oh I've never seen that big suitcase there before!') I keep fresh flowers in my room and more than one client has remarked on this, as something that makes them feel cared about. Some practitioners have more say than others about the contents of the room, depending on where they work. Some prefer to work in a neutral environment that reveals little and others feel more comfortable with personal items around. The physical cleanliness of the room is both an aesthetic thing and a health and safety issue. An emptied rubbish bin, a vacuumed carpet, clean treatment linen, fresh soap in the toilets, clean windows and dust free surfaces all look good but also contribute to a healthy treatment environment.

Rooms and energy

The energy of the room matters too because it effects our own energy bodies. Think about the difference between a busy station concourse and your bedroom. Close your eyes for a moment and imagine it. The energy in one is moving, in transition and busy. Depending who you are, you might find the station energy exciting and energising or you might feel depleted by it. Spaces also hold memories of events. I've never been there but I'm sure the energetic atmosphere in the concentration camps at Auschwitz must be overwhelming. We tend to feel good in places where healing has occurred, some holy buildings, and most natural habitats. If you ever go to Devon, visit the little church in Widdecombe-in-the-Moor. There's a quality of deep stillness in there that I've never found in all the big cathedrals full of secular tourist energy.

There are ways to look after our working space on an energetic level. Besides cleaning them energetically, we can dedicate them, borrowing ideas from ancient rituals. All religious traditions have practices which delineate the secular world from the spiritual – worship usually takes space in a building dedicated to that purpose – as well as rituals that mark the beginning and end of worship.

CLEANSING RITUALS

To cleanse the room's energy you can use incense, water, a candle flame, or a room spray (there are several on the market designed not to hide bad odours, or make your room smell like a springtime forest, but to settle energy). Starting in one corner, it doesn't matter which, wave the incense/flame around or sprinkle some water, lightly. Move along the wall to the next corner then in a complete circuit around the room. Hold in your intention some thought like 'I am cleaning my room' or 'I am purifying this space' – whatever feels right to you.

Another technique for settling the energy in a room is to use the four elements. Find something that represents air (examples: a feather, a picture of wind blowing through trees, a model of a bird), something for water (a picture of the sea, a small bowl of water), something for fire (a tea light in a holder, picture of a bonfire, a dragon, or a sunset) and something for earth (some salt in a saucer, a little flowerpot of earth, a small rock). Place one item in each corner of the room. Purists might say you have to put air in the east, water in the west and so on, but I don't think it really matters. Leave the objects in place as long as you need. If you are sensitive, you might feel the difference in the energy straight away. Things should settle down after an hour or so.

The client contract

Another boundary of the therapeutic relationship is the contract between the practitioner and the client that states what will happen, when, where and how, what the result might be and how much this service will cost. The contract sets a limit on the interaction; it states what will and what will not happen and draws the line between a professional relationship and any other kind.

Early on in my career I went to a supervisor called Rosalind. We sat on cushions in her living room surrounded by plants, candles and mirrors. It all seemed a bit magical to me. She was a good supervisor and I respected her. She listened well, made helpful suggestions and seemed to understand my difficulties. At the end of the hour I'd pay her and then she'd make us both a cup of tea and we'd chat for another half hour or so, about her son, her problems with her ex-husband, or she'd show me round her garden. At the time I felt flattered at being taken into her confidence, but also a bit uncomfortable. Much later, long after we'd said goodbye and I'd moved on, I realised I was very angry with her. She'd failed to be clear about our contract, hadn't acknowledged the power imbalance in our relationship and had assumed that it was fine for me to switch from supervisee to 'friend' just like that.

There are two aspects to the contract made between practitioner and client; the part that is explicit and the part that is assumed. So, when I describe how I work to a client and discuss terms with her, we're talking about information that is clearly communicated. But both of us also have assumptions about how the other will behave that don't get mentioned, and may not even be conscious. I'll assume that she's told me the truth about any medical conditions and that she can afford to pay me. She'll assume that I am qualified to do the treatment I'm offering and that I won't harm her in any way. She'll also assume that I'll stick to the same terms that I've laid out for her. So, if I say I'll see her at ten o'clock, this implies that I will be there at ten. These are reasonable sorts of expectations to have and we won't feel the need to discuss them. When the implicit terms aren't respected, things go wrong.

My friend Gini, for example, saw a bereavement counsellor after her mother died. 'She was a young woman, very nice, but she was always late. I felt as if she was always rushing from one place to another and I wasn't really that important.' She couldn't trust the counsellor and stopped going.

Contracts and the law

Every time you take on a new client the agreement you make is a legal contract. When you say, over the phone, 'I can see you at five o'clock for a reflexology treatment. It will cost £30', and the client agrees to the offer of treatment and to pay the price for it, a legal contact has been made. Basically, this means that one party offers the services at a price and the other accepts the terms and agrees to pay the price. The promises can be verbal or written down – both are equally binding in law, and they do not have to be written by lawyers in legal language. Paying for the goods in your basket at the supermarket is an example of contract law, as are buying a theatre ticket or paying for a car service.

There are three elements to a legal contract, all equally important. A lot of misunderstanding and client dissatisfaction can be avoided if practitioners pay good attention to all of them. There must be an offer, an acceptance and an agreed fee. For a complementary therapist in private practice, this means that the client knows the nature of the services you are offering, and how much they cost, and accepts both. Although this sounds very simple, a lot does depend on clarity of communication. The terms of the contract must be clear and unequivocal and the client must agree to them.

ISSUES TO CONSIDER WHEN MAKING CONTRACTS WITH CLIENTS

- People under the influence of alcohol or drugs, and those 'not in sound mind' may not be in a position to understand or agree to a contract.

- If you work with people under the age of 18, you may need the consent of a parent or guardian.

- Some practitioners sell gift vouchers for their treatments, and in this case, the contract is still made with the client who turns up for the treatment, even though the payment was from the person who bought the voucher.

- Practitioners who work in NHS settings don't have legal contracts with their clients. This is a complicated situation because the contract in law is between the practitioner and the NHS. However, it is still good practice to describe the nature of the treatment and obtain the client's acceptance, even when there is no direct payment.

- If you rent rooms in a clinic or health centre and operate as a self-employed practitioner the contract you make with your clients is the same, legally, as if you were working in private practice. If the centre employs you, the legal situation is much more complicated. But it is still your responsibility to make a clear agreement with the client and obtain acceptance.

Your client contract
This exercise is designed for therapists in private practice, but may be helpful to those who work elsewhere as an exercise in communication. Write your answers to the following questions.

1. What information do you give on the phone or by e-mail before meeting and what do you ask the client?

2. What do you say in the first session about the treatment, yourself or your terms?

3. What written information, if any, do you give to clients?

4. How do you know that the client has both understood and agreed to your terms?

Then consider your answers in the light of the following questions:

1. Do you communicate clearly how much a treatment costs, how and when payment should be made, your cancellation policy and length of a session?

2. Do you ask about a client's previous experience of your therapy, or what he expects from the treatment?*

3. Do you communicate clearly about possible duration of treatment, i.e. how many sessions the client might need to commit to or, where this is unclear, make this explicit?

4. Are you clear about possible outcomes, without giving absolute promises? Do you discuss possible adverse effects?

5. Do you recommend alternative therapies, including visiting a medical practitioner, if you think this might be more beneficial for the client?

6. Do you sum up the agreement reached during the session, and ask for the client's agreement? For example: 'Your lower back is hurting, your energy levels are low, and you've had some digestive trouble. As we discussed, I'm going to massage your back, buttocks, legs, working to relax your muscles, and do some energy holds on your tummy. Is that all right?'

7. Do you discuss confidentiality, and possible reasons to break it, e.g. to inform a medical health practitioner that you are seeing his patient, or to liaise with a specialist consultant?

8. Do you ask permission, or inform the client about record keeping?

9. Do you inform the client about your qualifications, professional organisation, and the code of conduct you adhere to, if asked?

---

* Your treatment may be a standard one given to all clients with little variation, like on-site chair massage, or it may be specific to the client's requirements, like homeopathy. The treatment may involve only one complementary therapy or may be a combination of two, or even three, for example an acupuncture treatment with a shoulder massage and some healing. Clients vary in their experience and knowledge of complementary therapy. A sophisticated user does not need to be given information about, say, what a reflexology session entails, how it works and the effect it might have, but someone new to the therapy does. Ideally, all of this needs to be spelt out and agreed to.

Personal boundaries

Each of us has a space around our bodies that we feel, on some unconscious level, is ours, and when another person comes into that space, especially if they enter without invitation, or suddenly, unexpectedly, our reactions let us know that something unpleasant, something not OK, has occurred. This is our personal space boundary. Unlike the physical boundary of a room, this is not a fixed space but one that expands or contracts depending on our environment, who we are with, our health and how tired we are. It is also partly determined by the culture that we grew up in.

When we move toward or touch another, our personal space merges with theirs. As practitioners we are responsible for monitoring our own personal space boundaries as well as having sensitivity and respect for those of our clients. If I am sitting too close to a client, my body sends out signals that interfere with my ability to focus. If I'm attuned, I notice this and move my chair but I'm also wondering if the signals are emanating from the other person. Am I too far into her space? Is my nervous system resonating with hers at this moment? Unless this is part of the work we're doing, and I'm negotiating with her about touch, or helping her discover her own personal space boundaries, I won't need to make this explicit. If I move, and create more space between us, we can both relax a little and breathe more easily.

Working with personal space

We take it for granted that if a client has agreed to treatment from us, particularly bodywork, that we have permission to move into his personal space. And on one level we do, of course, but that doesn't mean that he feels comfortable about it. The following exercises are designed to develop your own sense of comfort and discomfort around personal space, but they apply to any sort of personal boundary. They are also very useful to teach to clients. I've borrowed the terms 'this is OK' and 'this is not OK' as umbrella terms for comfort, ease, liking, and their opposites, from Antonio Damasio, who writes about the role that these bodily sensations play in our survival in his book *The Feeling of What Happens* (2000). He describes consciousness as the interface between our perceptions of the outside world as it is at this moment and our perception of our internal world as it is at this moment. A moment of core consciousness arises when I'm aware of all the stimuli from the environment meeting all those from my internal body state and I evaluate this mixture, at the very simplest level, as good for me or not good for me, and take steps to stop whatever is causing discomfort or stay with or increase that which feels good. We can access this sort of awareness through mindfulness practice, but most of the time our attention is caught by the loudest, fastest, brightest, most demanding information around or inside us. As human beings, we rarely allow ourselves moments of pure presence but bring our incredible ability to sort, contrast, compare, encode and make sense of information to any one moment of our existence.

Exercises to discover your own 'this is not OK' signal

When you can identify and recognise your own 'this is not OK' signals, you have an internal marker that can help you identify when something is not right in an interpersonal relationship, therapeutic or otherwise. We talk about gut instincts, and indeed, our guts do signal to us how our body is responding to any given situation. The lining of the small intestine, the yards of digestive tubing that lie coiled in a nest in the belly, produce more serotonin, the feel-good neurochemical, than the brain. Guts are a source of emotional responses.

✍ Exercise to map your personal space, using your 'this is not OK' signal

You need to do this one with a partner in a room that's large enough to move around in easily. Find a clear space in the room, and sit on a chair in the middle. Ask the other person to move to the edge of the space. Sit quietly for a moment, come into your body, let your breathing settle and do whatever you usually do to centre yourself, until you feel comfortable in your body. Then ask the other person to walk slowly towards you, keeping your attention in your body, and your physical sensations. There will be a moment when your inner sensations change, as the other enters your physical space. Ask him or her to stop, and repeat the exercise from another angle. So, if he or she came towards you from the front, try it again from the side, or behind. In fact, if you tried it from all angles, and drew a mark on the floor each time you said stop, you'd be able to see the shape of your own personal space.

But the point of this exercise is also to discover your 'this is not OK' signal. Here's a list of somatic responses you may have felt; there isn't a right or wrong response to this, each of us having our own particular signals. See if any apply to you:

- tight jaw
- clenched hands
- butterflies in your tummy
- change in breathing rate
- shallow breathing
- holding your breath
- tight shoulder muscles

- adrenaline surge
- increased heart rate
- nausea
- toes curled under.

There may be accompanying thoughts, such as

- Oh no.
- Go away.
- Stop.
- I don't like this.
- This isn't nice.

It isn't always fight or flight

Of course, what we're describing here are all signals of the fight or flight response, signs that we are becoming alert to the possibility of danger and need to prepare physically for the event. But there are other universal situations that also provoke a 'this is not OK' response, with corresponding physical sensations, which are not to do with excitement or danger.

Read through the following scenarios, pausing after each one to notice your inner physical sensations and emotional response.

1. A plate of raw liver has been given to you. Notice the dark red colour, the shiny surface, and the shape of the meat. Pick up a piece, feel how smooth and slippery it is, then take a mouthful.

2. You are having an aromatherapy massage. The smell of the oils is delicious, as is the sensation of the practitioner's hands on your back. But the room is very cold, and there's no extra heating.

3. You've woken up with a terrible hangover.

4. It's your birthday, and everyone in your house (if you live with others) acts as if it's an ordinary day. They've all forgotten. You check your e-mails, finding nothing. You wait for the post, thinking there might be a card but there are none.

All your responses to these little scenarios are your body's way of communicating about events that are bad for you, and that, if you persist, will eventually compromise your ability to survive as a living organism. If we didn't have inbuilt mechanisms to recognise food that was bad for us (although some people may eat raw liver, I suppose), or when we're too cold, dehydrated or poisoned, or devices that alert us to our needs for other people, we wouldn't have got far as a race.

✍ **Exercise to explore personal emotional boundaries with a client**
It's not just our physical space that we need to monitor when we work with people but also our emotional space. Now on the whole, people respect each other's emotional space but there are cultural differences, and some people just don't know when to stop!

Read through the following questions as if they were being asked by a client and notice how comfortable, or not, you feel. I know it depends on the person and the circumstances, but in general, you may find that there are some matters that you wouldn't mind sharing with clients and others that are definitely off limits.

1. Can I give you a hug?
2. Do you like your work?
3. Were you abused as a child?
4. Can I pay you next time I come?
5. Do you have massage/reflexology/see a homeopath regularly yourself?
6. Do you smoke/drink/do drugs?
7. Do you ever get turned on during a treatment?
8. Have you got children?
9. Can I give you a kiss?
10. Do you ever get fed up with your work?
11. Will you come to my birthday party?
12. Are you married?
13. Is it all right if I bring my dog in?
14. Do you like doing this?
15. How long have you been qualified?
16. Come for a drink with me some time?
17. Are you insured?
18. Do you do extras?
19. What are you doing on Saturday?
20. Do you earn a lot of money doing this therapy?

Most practitioners that I have talked with about these difficult kinds of questions agree that the ones to do with professional practice, such as 'How long have you been qualified?', feel acceptable, because the client is asking for information that he is entitled to have. Questions about the practitioner's personal life generally feel unacceptable, but also create a sense of curiosity. Why is this person asking me this? Is she just making conversation? Maybe she doesn't know the 'rules' of this sort of relationship. Maybe she does and needs, for whatever reason, to test them out. Some of these questions, which seem very inappropriate, may be someone's way of ascertaining how you will react to certain things. If you have had a similar experience, you may be more understanding and less judgemental. Questions about abuse, alcohol and drugs use or parenthood may mask an uncertainty about how much to disclose. Or there may be other reasons behind the question. One simple way to find out is to say 'That's an odd/interesting/strange question. Why do you ask?' Another is to deflect the question. 'Do I earn a lot of money? Well, you know what my fee is!'

Over the years I have been asked most of these questions, and find it helps to have standard responses, a phrase that I can retrieve automatically when my personal boundaries get pushed. I don't want to sit with my mouth open wondering what to say. So, for example, when a client suggests meeting for coffee, I might say, 'Thank you, that's a really kind offer but I'm afraid I don't socialise with clients'. If I think someone is just pushing boundaries I'll say, 'Good question, but, you know, that's my personal business'. These work for me, but might sound false or too formal for you. Read through the questions in the above exercise again, and see if you can find some standard responses that feel comfortable for you, things you could say with integrity, using language that suits you.

When the client's personal and emotional space isn't respected

The following are all true stories demonstrating lack of respect or sensitivity for personal and emotional space. In the first, the boundary of the professional relationship was blurred, and in the second two, the professional contract was broken.

My friend Julia has had a number of therapists who had flexible or unclear boundaries. Eventually she found someone who took these things very seriously. In the first session Julia said to her new therapist 'I don't want to know anything about you' – and seven years on she still doesn't, and that's exactly how she wants it. The most confusing experience prior to this was with a counsellor called Deirdre. They had a contract for one hour of counselling followed by one hour of massage, on a regular basis. The practitioner's flirtatiousness encouraged Julia to think there could be something between them, and she developed quite an attraction to Deirdre, and found herself becoming sexually excited during the massages. When Julia told her about her excitement, Deirdre acted as if she hadn't heard. After the therapy/massage ended, Deirdre became a friend, and socialised with Julia, still giving mixed messages about the possibility of an intimate relationship until Julia found herself so confused and upset she had to stop seeing her. This was a practitioner who had been very unclear about her own personal boundaries.

Marko was a trainer and practitioner for a bodywork organisation. He was charismatic, very gifted and completely unboundaried. I heard this story from Ann, a student on one of his trainings. She was also having individual treatments with him as a course requirement. One day when she arrived at his house for her session he answered the door, saying that he was running a bit late, and could she wait in the living room? There was already someone there, wrapped in a blanket and recovering from her treatment with Marko. When Ann finally saw him, nearly an hour late, he remarked that he didn't know what was happening, but everyone seemed to be going into their early birth stuff that day. Ann lay down, promptly went into her birth issues and got off the couch in deep shock. She arrived home two hours later and had to cancel the rest of her day's plans in order to recover. Afterwards, she reflected to me, she felt that Marko had been irresponsible. He was on a roll, enjoying the powerful impact of his work that day without due regard to the wishes and safety of his clients. He wasn't ensuring that people were safe to leave after their session with him, he wasn't sticking to time and people had to wait.

Jim was a shiatsu practitioner who I'd been seeing for a while. One particular day I gave my name to the clinic receptionist, as usual, and sat down to wait. The time of my appointment came and went. After another ten minutes I went up to the desk and the receptionist buzzed Jim's room, to discover he wasn't even in the building. She contacted him on his mobile and he explained that he'd been called to an emergency and could I make another appointment. No worry, I said, I'd go shopping. Actually, I felt pretty hurt and upset. Why hadn't he remembered my appointment? Why hadn't he even bothered to call the clinic to let them know? If I mattered that little to him, did I really want to go on seeing him? The answer was no. Jim lost a client that day.

When boundaries overlap: dual relationships

I was effleuraging John's back and he was chatting about the weather and the new parking regulations in his street, when he announced that he and Dennis were separating. He'd been seeing someone else and their relationship was over. My effleuraging hand froze and I felt the shock reverberate through my system. John and Dennis were both massage clients, attending weekly for three years, John to alleviate the stress from his high profile, high powered job as a city consultant and Dennis to manage a recurring low back problem. They were a committed couple and had been about to buy a second home by the sea. In addition, John had recently been diagnosed human immunodeficiency virus (HIV) positive and in my mind I'd begun to plan how to adapt my treatments to help him. Being a practical sort of person, some would say controlling, John had decided that it might be helpful for Dennis to 'talk to me', if I were willing, knowing that I also practised as a psychotherapist.

This posed several dilemmas. What was I to do for the best? First, I had to acknowledge my reactions to the news. I was fond of them, shocked by the suddenness of the news of their separation, and concerned for them both. I was pulled between wanting to support Dennis emotionally and John physically, with his altered health status. Next I needed to consider the situation wearing my professional hat. If I continued to see them both, would Dennis feel free to really express his feelings about John? How would we negotiate a change in our contract, from massage to counselling? Would it be unprofessional of me to stop seeing John at this point? Were there ethical issues to do with confidentiality?

In the end I talked with Dennis and we agreed to a short-term counselling contract to help him through the crisis. I said goodbye to John, who understood the confidentiality issues, and referred him to a colleague who specialised in treating people who were HIV positive.

This story illustrates the difficulties that arise when there are overlapping boundaries. Traditional psychoanalysis attempts to keep the therapeutic relationship as free as possible from external 'contamination' by keeping the boundaries very tight, in the same way that a scientist tries to control as many variables as possible in a research experiment, so that the hypothesis being tested is as free as possible from other influences. Real life and the therapeutic relationship inevitably and sometimes unavoidably overlap. Sometimes the overlapping might be trivial and unimportant but in other situations there may be considerable discomfort, for the practitioner or the client or both. Sometimes the overlapping is chosen, as when we knowingly agree to treat someone we know in another capacity, like a friend, and sometimes it happens inadvertently, like discovering that a client is on the management team of an organisation where you've applied to work.

Does it matter that the boundaries of the therapeutic relationship might overlap with another sort of relationship? This is a very complex issue. On the one hand, we are real people as well as complementary therapy practitioners and we do have lives outside the treatment room. If we let ourselves be imprisoned by our professional selves, some of our authenticity gets lost. If some of our outside life finds its way in to the treatment room our clients get to learn that we, too, are fallible and capable of mistakes or ordinary human frailty. I once had a little grey cat who would hide under a chair, unknown to me, and emerge in the middle of a session. Some clients loved it when this happened, others were indignant that another little being was claiming my attention, in their time. But given that the relationship between practitioner and client is a very important factor in the success of a treatment, I would argue that too much discomfort on the part of the practitioner or the client, whether from difficulties with dual roles or too much 'real life' getting into the treatment room, could interfere with a good outcome.

The Acupuncture Council's Code of Professional Conduct (item 25) says:

> You may sometimes find yourself called upon to treat a relative or someone who you consider a friend. There is no harm in this provided that clear boundaries are kept between the social and professional relationship.

Compare this with the British Medical Association's (BMA 2004) guidelines:

> Doctors are sometimes asked to treat their families or other people close to them. There are clearly some cases, such as in emergencies, in which such action would be resonable, but as a general rule it should be avoided. A confusion of roles can develop and doctors can find it hard to keep the right emotional distance... They may have conflicts of interest or be erroneously perceived as having such conflicts.

But it also mentions that 'It is hard to lay down an absolute rule: it makes sense for a doctor to treat minor ailments, or take emergency action where necessary'.

Although some complementary therapy professional codes of conduct might hint at the difficulties and emphasise the fact that it is the practitioner's responsibility to be clear about the difference between professional and personal boundaries, none are as clear as the BMA that it is inadvisable and there aren't any hard and fast rules for dealing with dual relationships. The main thing is for us to be aware of them.

Dual relationships in the context of training

Complementary therapy trainings are experiential as well as theoretical and students are required to receive the therapy that they are learning. Some of this takes place as practice sessions with peers; massage, shiatsu, Reiki, acupuncture, osteopathy and craniosacral students practise on each other in and out of class. But often there is a requirement to receive treatment from an experienced practitioner as well. This enables the student to learn about good practice, to experience the difference between an established practitioner and a novice and to have someone available to 'mop up' mistakes made during practice, or deal with the emotional issues that arise during the course. None of us who've been through, or taught on, professional trainings would deny that the experiential part brings personal issues to the forefront for students. If the experienced practitioner assigned to, or chosen by, the student is separate from the training, there are no overlapping boundaries and the student can feel free to express whatever she needs. However, if the practitioner is also a course tutor, and, even more difficult, a tutor who is responsible for assessing the student, might she not feel more restricted talking about personal things? Some training organisations have become aware of the potential difficulty for a student in dealing with the dual relationship of a tutor and assessor also being a personal practitioner, and stipulate a clear demarcation between the two.

Dual relationships and your comfort levels

How comfortable are you working with dual relationships? It may be something you never encounter, if, for example, you only work with a specific population such as elderly clients in hospital care. It may be something you do all the time, if you are the only complementary therapist in a small community. But as an interesting exercise, go through the following list and spend a moment asking yourself honestly how comfortable you feel working with each type of client. Try using your 'this is OK/not OK' signals.

As a practitioner, how comfortable would/do you feel if your client is:

- a colleague

- a friend

- your hairdresser

- one of your students (if you teach your therapy)

- a family member

- a famous television personality

- the partner of another of your clients

- someone you also supervise.

As a client yourself, how comfortable would/do you feel having treatment from:

- a colleague

- a friend

- one of your students

- a family member

- one of your teachers

- an ex-client who has trained as a complementary therapist.

Suggestions for dealing with overlapping boundaries

Remember, there are no right or wrong ways of dealing with these issues, and it is your job to take responsibility for them, not your clients'.

1. If you are aware of overlapping relationships with a client, consider whether it is one you are comfortable with. If not, and you think that your discomfort might get in the way of your professionalism, refer the person to someone else.

2. Consider the client's interests. Might he feel uncomfortable with an overlapping relationship? Discuss it with him. Acknowledge that these things can feel difficult.

3. Are there issues of confidentiality that might create tension in either the working relationship, or your social relationship, for either of you? For example, if treating a family member means gaining access to very personal or sensitive information that no one else in the family was aware of, you'd be under obligation, through professional confidentiality, to keep a secret. Let's take a couple of extreme examples: would you feel comfortable knowing an uncle was a cocaine user, or a teenage niece was pregnant, and only you knew about it?

When boundaries get broken

There's a difference between a boundary crossing and a boundary violation. The first kind is repairable and, if dealt with sensitively, may even strengthen the therapeutic relationship. The second is more serious, leads to a breakdown in relationship, the loss of a client and could even be the basis of a grievance claim from the client to your professional organisation.

Examples of boundary crossing:

- When I failed to leave enough time to get to work, or was held up in traffic, and found the client waiting on the doorstep.

- The occasion that I called a client by her partner's name instead of her own.

- The times that I have let a session overrun without asking the client's permission to do so. (I think it's not uncommon for practitioners working in private practice to do this, but be warned! I heard about a case in the USA of a psychotherapist being sued in court by a client for consistently running over time and not charging for it.)

- Letting a client hug me when I didn't really want to be hugged.
- Forgetting to pull down the blind on the window before starting a treatment.

Examples of boundary violations within the therapeutic context:

- When I hugged a client, realising too late that it was quite inappropriate and more to do with my needs than hers. She didn't come back.
- When a male massage student removed the towel so far that he exposed the breasts of an elderly woman client, who only wanted her neck massaged.
- When a practitioner asked a client, who thought she had come for a Reiki healing, to undress. The practitioner had decided the client needed massage but hadn't consulted or informed her.
- A reflexologist who rang his female clients at home to ask if they'd enjoyed their sessions.

Some boundary violations are obvious cases of negligence or misconduct on the part of the practitioner, but not all. To some extent how the client experiences the break (error, mistake) determines whether the incident is a violation or not. For example, if I am massaging a colleague who I know has no issues about his body or nudity, I won't bother to tell him when I am about to remove the towel to massage his gluteals. However, if I were to act in the same way with a woman who had recently been raped, and wanted to receive massage to repair the emotional damage to her body, I would be making a gross and insensitive boundary violation. Reactions to boundary violations may be delayed, and emerge after the session is over, so the practitioner may not hear about it until the next time she sees the client. Or she may never know about it, if the person who's experienced the violation chooses not to confront but to leave. Or until she gets a letter from the client's solicitor.

Complaints about complementary therapy practitioners are still relatively rare. Witness, (known as POPAN, the Prevention of Professional Abuse Network until November 2005) is an organisation 'dedicated to helping people who have been abused by health and social care workers and working to prevent abuse'. Only about 5–10 per cent of the people they help have been abused by health professionals compared to counsellors and psychotherapists, but they do point out that this may be because they have a much higher profile in that arena. But they (and other researchers in the area of professional abuse) point out that 70 per cent of their clients who experience boundary violations within a therapeutic relationship were sexually, physically or emotionally abused in childhood (see www.popan.org.uk). There are many arguments as to why this might be so, one of which being that a person who has experienced traumatic or multiple boundary violations is going to be highly sensitised to such occurrences, and will be more affected by them.

Examples of boundary crossings outside the therapeutic context

The scenarios above are all ones that occur within the framework of the therapeutic relationship and, as such, can be dealt with, discussed and apologised for at the time they occur. But there are some scenarios that we have no control over, where real life meets the therapeutic relationship head on — situations when you aren't wearing your professional hat and acting as such. How would you feel about these?

- Naked, you meet a client in the sauna.

- You have a heated altercation at the supermarket checkout and swear at the cashier. As you leave, you notice a client in the queue, watching you.

- You see your acupuncturist/homeopath/shiatsu practitioner having a heated altercation at the supermarket checkout and swearing at the cashier.

- You and your wife/husband have a messy divorce that gets into the local paper. A client comes in with a copy of the paper in her bag.

- You're having dinner in a restaurant when a client comes over and starts chatting.

- You discover that your Reiki healer/reflexologist/chiropractor is having a secret affair with your (married) best friend.

What to do? Remember, it is your responsibility to deal with the situation. I did once meet a client in the sauna and gave her the chance to express her feelings about it in our next session by suggesting that it must have been strange, meeting me like that. This indicated that I was aware it could have been awkward, but also gave her the choice to follow up or not. She could say no or talk about it at length. I wasn't jumping to any conclusions about her response to seeing me naked. If, and only if, she had expressed shock or dismay I might have apologised, or asked her how we should go about things if it ever happened again.

A rough guideline might be:

- Name it. Find a way to mention – lightly – the incident.

- Give the client the opportunity to discuss it.

- If she doesn't want to, respect this and move on.

- If she wants to talk, let her and just listen.

- Empathise (yes, that must have been difficult for you), apologise (I'm so sorry that you witnessed that) or mirror (I can hear that you're quite upset) as appropriate.

Clients who break boundaries

Of course, it isn't just us, the professionals, who break boundaries. Our clients do it too. We've probably all had the person who arrives ten minutes early or late, misses appointments, and cancels at the last minute on a regular basis. It may be that this person's life is chaotic, or he has chronic difficulties with time keeping, but it may just be that he doesn't understand the rules. Then there are the clients who, no matter how professional we are, treat us like their best friend. People who ask inappropriate questions about our personal lives. Or make phone calls at all hours of the night. We tend to assume that people who come to see us will, at least, have been to a doctor and be capable of extrapolating from that situation to this. Or have had interviews for work, or seen a visit to a complementary practitioner during an episode of soap on television. Some things about the interaction we take so much for granted that it never occurs to us to mention them.

Here's a true example. I was a bit shocked to notice that a client didn't shut the door when she used the toilet. The second time it happened I realised that it wasn't a forgetful oversight but that she just didn't know the rules, and was, perhaps, acting in a clinic setting in the same way she did at home, without recognising how inappropriate this was. So I mentioned to her that, because there were men in the building, she might feel more comfortable if she shut the door and locked it next time she used the toilet.

There's a greater likelihood that certain kinds of clients will mis-understand the 'rules' of the therapeutic relationship and therefore break boundaries or behave inappropriately. These people aren't messing us about or being 'bad' clients; they need extra guidance and help. The implicit norms of behaviour tend to be white, British and middle class. Anyone who doesn't belong in these categories or hasn't had the opportunity to learn the norms is disadvantaged. This includes clients from varied cultural backgrounds, particularly non-English-speaking ones, those with learning difficulties and maybe some with mental health problems. Boundary testing may also be a feature with people who have been abused, as a way of testing you and the safety of the situation. Do you mean what you say? Are you consistent? Does no mean no? Again, this is someone not being bad, but trying to ascertain if you are a safe person.

When a boundary break can be a good thing

And finally, every once in a while, a boundary break can be just the right thing to happen. Amelie is someone I'd been seeing for years for massage, and during that time she too had trained as a massage practitioner, and then as a chiropractor. One day when she came for her treatment I'd twisted an ankle quite badly and was limping. She asked all about it, how it happened, we wondered together which ligaments might have been damaged, and after her session ended she asked if I had another client straight away, then said, 'Put your foot up here.' And held my ankle for five minutes or so. Normally I'd feel very uncomfortable about such a complete reversal of role, but I didn't at that moment with Amelie. 'I can feel the shock where you fell, right up to your knee' she said, and my ankle certainly felt better for her mini-treatment. Thinking about it afterwards, there was one important factor that contributed to it being a positive experience. By allowing her to look after me I was acknowledging her as an equal, as a professional in her own right and letting her demonstrate her care and concern for me. It would have been churlish and wounding of me to refuse her healing.

Disclosure

Disclosure refers to the information about our personal selves to which we allow clients access. It doesn't mean our thoughts about the client's issues, treatment options or our reactions to things that occur during the session. These are all part of the professional relationship; even though they are more about us than the client, they are oriented to the client and his or her well being. If we remember the idea of a boundary as a container, then disclosure refers to the matter that we, the practitioner, put into the container, that is about us as human beings.

Some personal information is obvious as soon as we meet the other person and we can't hide it. Sex, age, skin colour, body type and some aspects of physical ability (wearing glasses or using a wheelchair, for example) are obvious. Our accents may give away information about our background and our clothes, if we don't wear a work uniform of some kind, give messages about the extent we care about our appearance, our personal style or lack of it, where we shop and so forth. Of course we can't know whether or not our clients interpret the messages that all these things say about us correctly, but they all convey personal information that can't be easily hidden. How much we choose to tell clients about ourselves, to disclose deliberately, is something to consider because of the manner in which disclosure affects the boundaries of the relationship. The more a client knows about your personal values, your family and social life, the more the relationship may begin to feel like a friendship. More intimacy, trust and liking for each other can lead to a blurring of the boundary between a professional and a personal relationship. A common difficulty for students on massage trainings, who do swaps with each other, or practise on family and friends, occurs when the treatment is over and the reason for being together ends, but there is also another kind of connection which requires a cup of tea, or a chat about the family and takes up time and presents the student with the dilemma of how to tell someone who is not really a client that it's time to leave. Likewise the professional who offers cups of tea after a treatment, and doesn't say clearly when it is time to leave, is creating an unclear boundary.

I think there may be a tendency among complementary therapists to treat clients in a friendly manner as a reaction to the perceived, stereotypical (and, these days, inaccurate) image of the cold impersonal medical health professional who was interested in symptom not person. We are holistic, we treat the whole person, we are interested in his life, and in her perception of her illness and so we think we can be more relaxed.

It might be worth examining the role that disclosure plays in your therapeutic relationships, not because there is anything wrong with being a human being rather than a robot, but because the more conscious we are of our behaviour and how it might enhance or detract from the overall purpose of our work, the better. There are several factors to consider: the nature of the information about yourself that you share, how often you do it, who with and, most importantly, for what purpose.

What type of information do you disclose?

To some extent this will depend on how open or private a person you are. Recently I knew of two colleagues who had similar family crises. Both of them were caring for an elderly parent who was dying. One told all his clients while the other told none of hers. The practitioner who disclosed is a very open person, who believes in honesty and being real with his clients. The practitioner who didn't is a very private person who needed her work as a refuge from her feelings about her personal situation. Two very different ways of handling a situation, neither of them right or wrong, but each right for that person at that time.

Do you talk with clients about:

- Family and everyday life such as your partner, parents, children, their schooling, where you live, what car you drive, your pets, where you go on holiday, which films you've seen.

- Your values and beliefs such as who you vote for, your spiritual path and practices, your opinions on current affairs.

- Your personal health history, including therapies that you've tried, operations, or medications you've used, your current state of health.

- Your other clients.

Which clients do you disclose to?

- All your clients equally.

- Only some types of clients.

- Clients who are more like you (roughly the same age, background, the same sex).

- Clients who are less like you (different sex, age, background).

When I was thinking about this question for myself, I started with the assumption that I treated everyone the same in this respect, but the more I considered it – I went through in my mind all the sessions I'd done that week and what I'd told to whom – I got quite a surprise. You might too.

How often do you disclose?

- As a matter of course, in most sessions, during the initial consultation and the treatment?

- Do you only offer personal information if a client asks you? If someone asks a question that is too personal, how do you deal with it? (Another colleague of mine has a good response to this one. He says, 'That's a good question. [Pause] And I'm not going to answer it'.)

- Regularly?

- Rarely?

What's the purpose of the disclosure?

This is probably the most important question. Does disclosure serve the relationship, or the client or both? Or does it create problems in terms of boundary maintenance? Not all clients want a friendly relationship with their practitioner. In fact, my friend Sara was very relieved to find a chiropractor who didn't talk at all, other than for professional purposes, because, having been to lots of different complementary therapists over the years, she was tired of the chatty, friendly approach, was beginning to find it intrusive and just wanted to have her treatment and be left alone.

- Do you disclose in order to build the relationship? For example, if someone arrives with a dripping umbrella, might you describe your journey in the rain as well?

- For educational reasons? If a client is wondering about trying a certain herbal remedy, would you talk about your own experience taking it, whether it worked for you, or where to find it?

- To help normalise a client's experience? For example, digestive rumblings during bodywork sessions embarrass many people. Might you say that you too used to feel like that, and it's normal to feel embarrassed?

- For your own purposes, because, for example, that's just the sort of person you are, or chatting helps you overcome nervousness?

Some legal aspects of the therapeutic relationship

The laws pertaining to complementary therapy provide a framework or boundary to the therapeutic relationship. They exist to protect our clients and us, provide guidelines for good practice and procedures for grievances.

When I started practising as a complementary therapist nearly 20 years ago, the general approach to clients was friendly, informal and trusting. The spectre of litigation hadn't raised its ugly head, and the only discussions about 'the law' i.e. police and the courts, were those to do with confidentiality, and circumstances in which the practitioner might decide, or be required, to pass on information about a client to another agency.

Things have changed a lot since then. David Balens, of the Balens insurance brokers, a firm that deals with many complementary therapies, writes in *Shiatsu Society News* (2004), that attempts by clients to claim compensation from practitioners is on the increase, as are allegations of sexual impropriety or assault. We live in an increasingly transparent, accountable and target orientated culture, and there are a number of laws that CAM therapists need to be acquainted with. Your professional code of conduct and ethics will overlap with these legal issues and some may incorporate them directly.

Client dissatisfaction can arise from number of sources, according to David Balens. These seem to fall into two categories. There are those arising from poor contractual agreements, such as a lack of clear information, paying too much or for too long for treatment, being given unrealistic expectations about outcome of treatment and not being consulted about treatment. The importance of making clear contracts is discussed in the section on boundaries in Chapter 1. The other kinds of dissatisfaction arise from failures in the therapeutic relationship, including feeling disrespected, embarrassed or misunderstood, or experiencing abuse from a practitioner.

What does the law have to do with anything that happens in private in our treatment rooms?

1. The therapeutic interaction takes places within a legal framework, which, ideally, supports the contractual relationship we make with a client, and protects the clients' rights.

2. Next, the laws pertaining to health and safety affect hygiene, use and disposal of materials, and handling of equipment and clients and the premises we work in.

3. The Freedom of Information and the Data Protection Acts impact on how we keep records, the sort of records we keep, and confidentiality.

4. We may be required to give written evidence for insurance purposes for accident claims. We may be required to appear in court, if, for example, an expert witness is required to give evidence in a case brought against a colleague for malpractice, or to give evidence in a coroner's court if a client commits suicide.

5. If a client makes a complaint, the matter should be dealt with first by the relevant complaints and disciplinary committee of the professional organisation, following their own complaints procedure. If the client feels that the complaint has not been dealt with effectively, he could then proceed with a legal complaint.

6. And finally, working with certain client groups, particularly those in recovery from chemical abuse, and users of the mental health system, may require knowledge of relevant legislation.

Malpractice and negligence

Complementary therapists are obliged to have public liability and malpractice insurance. What exactly constitutes malpractice? The law makes subtle and complex distinctions between different kinds of mistakes, malpractice and negligence, which depend to some extent on the degree of harm to the client.

Complementary therapists have duties of care to their clients that oblige them not to harm or damage but to use their skills to treat and care for them. This applies whether or not there is also a contractual arrangement. If a practitioner is negligent, she or he has failed to provide reasonable care and can be sued by the client, although the incidence of this happening is still very low. There's also a difference between a mistake, which is an unintentional failure of good practice such as forgetting the key to the cupboard where case notes are stored, and doing something that's a careless failure of minimum good practice that could harm a client, like, for example, knowingly treating clients with compromised immune functioning when you have an infection. Serious professional misconduct might include having sex with a client during a session, selling a client's story to the media or exchanging blows with a client.

Record keeping and confidentiality

Why keep records? A full medical history, together with indications and contraindications to your particular therapy, is needed for insurance purposes as well as your own reference. Records provide an aide-memoire to treatment given in sessions and note progress or changes in a client's condition. They are used when liaising with other professionals, and as evidence in case of a complaint. In this last instance, David Balens recommends that all communications with clients that concern contractual information, change of treatment and client consent are noted, including phone conversations, on top of keeping dated case notes, treatment records, correspondence with other professionals, and test results.

In some working situations complementary therapists may be part of a team, either of other practitioners working together with a client, or a team of practitioners from the same discipline who share clients. While it is always good practice to keep legible, clear notes, using appropriate technical terminology rather than your own subjective terms, this is particularly relevant where notes may be available to other practitioners.

The client's personal information, including name, address, occupation, contact details, GP, age, and next of kin, must be kept separately from all other notes. These, the treatment notes, contain the reason for seeking treatment, medical history, assessment and diagnosis, treatment given, changes noted and aftercare advice, and should not contain any information that could identify the client. This applies to notes kept electronically and hand written. All notes must be kept in a secure place. When the notes are not in use, people who have no need to see them should not have access to them. It is good practice to keep notes for seven years after treatment ends, or in the case of a child, for seven years after he or she turns 21. All practitioners who keep records of members of the public are required to register with the Data Protection Agency for a small annual fee.

Malpractice or not?

Think about the following scenarios and decide which might involve malpractice.

A receptionist at a health centre gives Aysha her notes to take in to the homeopath. She notices that the folder has her name, address and date of birth on the cover.

Mike is very surprised when his acupuncturist, having inserted all the needles, begins to massage his feet, instead of leaving him to rest, which is her usual practice.

When she leaves her reflexology session, Janet is a bit sleepy and trips over a loose paving stone in the street, breaking her leg.

Maura is a loving and compassionate healer and always kisses her clients on the cheek when they arrive and hugs them when they leave.

Jamie has to collect his children from school and drop them off at the child minder before starting his evening clinic. One afternoon, his youngest son is sick in the car, then the child minder isn't at home and by the time he's made other arrangements he's running an hour late and has several clients waiting for him.

Janet, her leg in plaster, seems to have fared the worst, compared to all the other clients. Who hasn't had to wait for their appointment or been hugged by a practitioner when they didn't particularly feel like it? Does it matter if a client's identifying information is on her notes and what's the matter with getting a bit of unexpected treatment? But let us assume that Janet's reflexologist had noticed her sleepy state, had given her a drink of water before she left and had told her to be careful. This practitioner had exercised her duty of care and the accident had happened on the street where this responsibility no longer operated. If Janet had tripped on a loose carpet in the clinic before leaving, her practitioner might be responsible for failing to meet health and safety requirements but, as it is, the accident was not her responsibility.

Aysha's homeopath contravenes the Data Protection Act by not separating her client's name, address and date of birth from her case notes. Mike's acupuncturist is possibly in breach of contract by changing the treatment option without consultation. Maura is using inappropriate or unwanted touch and could be accused of negligence on this count and Jamie is also in breach of contract by not turning up, albeit unintentionally.

4

Communication Skills

Birdsong is a chirp of meditative silence
Rendered in fluttered boughs, and I am still,
Very still, in philosophical light.
I am all ears in my waterside aviary.
My breath is poised for truth to whisper
From hidden invisibilities and the holiness
Venturesome little birds live with always...
(Douglas Dunn, 'The Year's Afternoon', 2000, p.3)

Listening

The speaker in this poem is taking three hours' respite from ordinary life, its schedules and demands, somewhere among trees and grass. He is so still that he 'sink[s] like a slow root'. The section above describes how he listens, mindfully and with total presence, for the truth to unfold. How often do we really listen, to our own inner voices, to the silence embedded in the noise around us, to hidden truths? How often do we really listen to another person when he talks? In everyday conversation, our minds race ahead, wanting to ask questions, add our bit to the story, agree or disagree. Half our attention is on the words that we're hearing and half on our response. There's an expectation that we will reply quickly, to keep the ball in the air, to prevent the dialogue from floundering. One of the basic listening exercises often used on training courses involves people getting into pairs, one to talk while the other just listens, without responding. Maybe you can remember the first time you ever had to do this exercise, and how hard it was to stop yourself from butting in. When it was your turn to talk, it may have seemed frightening or wonderful or both to have all of someone's attention on you, and you may have realised how rarely that happens.

It's a gift, to be listened to with quiet intention and total attention. I remember one of my teachers coming over to talk to me in a room packed with students trying out the technique he'd demonstrated earlier. As he sat down, I could almost see his focus shifting from wide range, encompassing the whole room, to settle down and in on me, like a powerful beam adjusted to close up. I knew I had his full attention and felt very moved by this. Another of my teachers used to say that all a good healer has to do is listen and get out of the way, and sooner or later, the client will tell you everything you need to know, including the answer to her own questions.

If you work with the body using touch, your hands will have learned how to listen to the tissues, or to energy flow. What would it be like to listen to the words a person says with the same sensitivity and single channel attention? Do you listen differently to your clients compared to how you listen to friends? I once asked a group of practitioners to do a listening exercise in pairs. They were all very experienced and I wondered if they could identify the difference between ordinary and professional listening. The brief was for the listener to listen to her partner first as if she were a friend and next with their practitioner hat on, as if they were listening to a client. Alice and her partner didn't find much difference. As Alice explained, listening professionally had helped her to become a good listener in any situation. However, when the exercise finished, Alice began chatting to her partner – interrupting, finishing sentences and so on, because special listening was no longer called for! Julie's partner described noticing something when Jane shifted from ordinary to professional listening, which was hard to describe but involved the intensity of Julie's focus. Julie herself spoke of ordinary listening being like hearing a list, or a story, whereas listening as a professional meant paying attention to the story but also to the patterns behind the words. The questions 'Who is this person?', 'Why is he telling me this?' and 'What is really being communicated here?' became as important as the immediate message in the words.

Good listening takes practice but it can make a big difference to our clients. None of us is used to being listened to well and yet we all have a huge need to be understood. Someone with confidence, the belief that he will manage to gain and maintain another person's attention and be able to say what he wants is more likely to get listened to. But what about those who lack such qualities? People who speak another language, children, people with disabilities and those who are just shy don't feel entitled to speak and be heard in the same way.

The first prerequisite for good listening is presence. It helps to be grounded and centred before you start to listen. It helps to take a deep breath and let go, with the out breath, of any preoccupations, thoughts or feelings of your own. They'll be there waiting if you still need to come back to them later on. Settle down and be present with the other person. The second important factor, while you are practising good listening, is to switch off your self listening, and to make your attention single channel, totally on the other person. I used to get quite anxious doing this, afraid that I'd forget what I wanted to say, or that nothing would come, or I'd forget what I was being told. Then I learned that it didn't matter, because the crucial part of the practice was the quality of the attention I could offer the person to whom I was listening. And eventually I learned to listen to myself and to the other person at the same time. The necessary factors are to be fully present, hearing how things are said as well as what is being said, noticing gestures, tone of voice and facial expressions and being aware of what is not said and is held back, under the surface.

Listening exercises

✍ Mindful listening

An easy exercise that can be done anywhere anytime. Take a few minutes when you won't be interrupted. You can do it on the bus, in bed, at the computer or washing the dishes. Stop whatever you are doing, settle down into yourself and listen to all the sounds around you. Traffic, voices, central heating noises, clocks ticking, planes overhead, birdsong, wind through leaves, whatever you hear, listen and let it go. Keep your attention relaxed, don't try too hard and, if your mind wanders, gently bring it back to the task in hand – mindful listening.

✍ Levels of listening

There are many ways to listen to what another person is saying. Here's an exercise to try listening on different levels. You'll need a recording of someone telling a story, something that you can listen to more than once. You could tape a radio interview, or go to an audio stories online website. Have writing materials to hand.

1. Play the story and listen to the content. Try to remember as much detail as you can. When it's finished, write down all you can remember.

2. Play it again, listening for the emotional content. What emotions are being talked about, or expressed directly? Make a note.

3. Play it again, this time listening with your guts. That's right, with your attention centred in your abdomen. Don't focus so hard on the words. When it's finished, write down what that felt like.

4. This time, centre your attention in your heart. When you're ready, switch on and listen again. What's it like to listen with your heart?

5. Finally, listen one more time for the message buried in the story. What do you think the storyteller is really trying to communicate? Write your comments.

✍ **Listening in everyday life**
You can practise listening on different levels in day-to-day conversations. Observe the ways that you usually listen to family, friends, colleagues, children or people in shops. Do you listen to everyone with the same degree of attention? How do you listen, and to what – content, feeling, the underlying message? Practise doing it differently. Try switching the focus from your mind to your heart, or listen to the emotional content rather than the words.

✍ **Listening to spirit**
Our ears are the physical organs that register the pattern of sound waves and convert them into neural patterns for our brains to interpret as noise, music, chatter or running water. If you work with the chakra system, you might like to try this exercise. Our throat chakra, the energetic communication centre, picks up information on a more subtle level. Sit quietly, settle into yourself and imagine that you have large conical structures, like old-fashioned ear trumpets, fanning out on each side of your head just below your ears that can collect and amplify the invisible truths hidden in the spaces between the sounds around you. Just wait, expect nothing and see what happens.

Listening and reflecting back

We give another person a sense of really being understood when we are able to state back what she has just said, and in our own words convey the feeling expressed, so that the speaker feels that it all came from her. This technique is sometimes called mirroring, because it is like holding a big mirror up to show someone her reflection. In everyday speech, someone might say 'Let me recap what you've just told me', which is another way of putting it. Here are some examples:

CLIENT: When my mother in law came to stay, everything changed. I think that's when my headaches got worse, yes, and I did my back in when I picked her up when she fell, and then I couldn't sleep well, for worrying about her at night, was she going to get up and wander around.

PRACTITIONER: Your headaches, sleeping difficulties and your back problems are all related to your mother in law living with you now?

CLIENT: I've got a rash on my legs, a red blotchy one, it doesn't itch but I'm worried because it's like the one my friend got when we were children, and his rash turned out to be an allergy to shellfish, which nearly killed him. He had prawns at his wedding reception and spent the first night of his honeymoon in the hospital. I'm getting married next month, see, and I don't want anything to go wrong.

PRACTITIONER: You're worried about your rash in case it turns out to be an allergic response to shellfish and you don't want your wedding to be spoilt?

CLIENT: When I first came to this country I was very glad to have escaped the war, and even though I don't have to fear for my life now, I know I'm safe, I still have days when I can't go out of the door and I just cry. I'm a grown man and I shouldn't be crying, I have to be strong for my wife.

PRACTITIONER: Even though you know you're safe in this country, there are times when you get very upset, and feel that you shouldn't.

Clear communication

We all know how to communicate clearly, don't we? Yes and no. In any verbal exchange between two people, there's the message that the speaker intends to convey and the message that the listener receives. If the communication is clear, these two messages are the same, and the listener hears and understands the meaning that the speaker wanted to get across. We tend to assume that this is happening whenever we have a conversation, take a case history or give a client instructions or advice. It can be quite startling when it's obvious that there's been a misunderstanding.

PRACTITIONER: [asking a client about the onset, he thinks, of a chronic arthritic condition] When did you first notice the pain in your joints?

CLIENT: [assuming the practitioner is asking about the recent flare up] Two nights ago.

If we can assume that there is always the chance that something can go amiss in the space between the words leaving one person's mouth and arriving at the ears, and then brain, of another then it behoves us to pay attention to our communication skills, to how we talk to others and how we listen to them. And to remember that the chance of a misunderstanding is increased if both people do not speak the same mother tongue, have any degree of hearing loss (very common the older we get), or have learning difficulties.

Factors that contribute to clear communication from the practitioner

VOICE

Brett Kahr, writing in a book called *What Works in Psychotherapy* (Ryan 2005), goes as far as to suggest that the warmth and general musicality of the practitioner's voice is a crucial, if underrated, factor in the therapeutic relationship.

> ...the patient will be deeply affected by our tone of voice, our accent, the volume of our voice, the pitch of our voice, its cadence, its flow, its presence, as well as by our sentence structure, our knowledge of grammar, and by the richness or paucity of our actual vocabulary. (p.10)

Although it is true that the practitioner's voice and all its variables are of more consequence in a talking therapy, I think there are points that are relevant for complementary therapists. For example, I have a naturally soft voice, which is an asset if I'm leading someone through a guided visualisation, but, as I discovered when working with a group of elders, problematic for people with hearing difficulties. I had to learn to speak up a bit, and to project my voice more than I was used to, without shouting. Deaf clients have taught me the importance of keeping my face out of shadow and turned towards the listener, and not covering my mouth with my hand, so that my lips are available for reading.

The volume, the speed of delivery and clarity of articulation matter if the speaker is to be understood. Rapid speakers may be hard to follow, while words paced too slowly risk sounding patronising, as if the speaker... is...talking...to...someone...who...is...not...very...bright. The tone, pitch and flow of speech convey other sorts of information that may affect the listener even when he can understand quite clearly what is being said. Consider the following sentences said with a sweet, gushing tone of voice, and then with a gentle, matter of fact tone. 'Some movements may feel a little uncomfortable. If I do something that is too painful, please let me know.'

Some of the variables to do with how we speak can be altered with very little effort when we become conscious of them – volume, speed, pitch – and some, like our accent, are fixed and more resistant to quick change, although some people who are naturally very empathetic take on the accents of people around them without even realising they are doing so. One way to create empathy in the relationship is to match those variables that you can to the listener's. Slowing or quickening the speed at which you talk or matching the pitch, volume or tone to the other person is a form of mirroring, like adopting the same body posture, and helps the client feel understood.

But if a client arrives upset, frightened or angry, or becomes so during a session, it wouldn't then be helpful to match your voice to hers and, if you did, it would probably make matters worse. Lowering your voice and speaking more slowly and more firmly may help to calm the other person, something many probably do naturally without even realising.

EYE CONTACT

Good eye contact means getting the right balance between making visual connection, staring and holding someone's gaze for too long. Good eye contact communicates sincerity and honesty, but most people are only comfortable with it for about three seconds. After that, it becomes too intimate, too familiar. There are cultural differences about the use of eye contact. For example, in the UK we say that someone who avoids eye contact is shifty, or has something to hide, but in Asia and Latin America, avoiding eye contact is a mark of respect.

CHOICE OF WORDS

There are two reasons why the sort of words you use, the length of sentences and how you phrase things matter: first, if what you say is too complicated, obscure or vague the message will be lost; and, second, if what you say is at odds with the client's frame of reference there'll be a mismatch and the difference between you will be highlighted rather than the similarity.

Using words that your client will understand helps to get the message across but should also be matched to her level of knowledge. If you say 'I'm going to palpate the medial edge of your gastrocnemius', 'I think your gallbladder meridian is unbalanced' or 'I'll find a remedy for the syphilitic miasm first' to a person who has never been near a complementary therapist in her life, you will be communicating gobbledygook, reinforcing the power imbalance between you and maybe alarming the client. If you didn't use these phrases when treating a fellow massage therapist, shiatsu practitioner or homeopath, on the other hand, you'd be failing to acknowledge the other's equal status as a professional. When a client has a limited grasp of English language it's best to avoid jargon and use everyday words. So choose terms that fit the listener's level of knowledge and ability to comprehend.

Matching the client's language demonstrates respect for the client's frame of reference and facilitates the working alliance. Adopting the words and phrases that the client uses to describe her experience, even if they are different from your own, fosters a sense of being understood. Read the two examples, to get a sense of this.

Practitioner asks client to describe her symptoms.

CLIENT: It's like someone was holding my guts and twisting them, down here at the bottom of my belly.

PRACTITIONER: You've got griping pains. What happens if you press your abdomen?

Practitioner asks client to describe her symptoms.

CLIENT: It's like someone was holding my guts and twisting them, down here at the bottom of my belly.

PRACTITIONER: And what happens to that sensation of twisting if you press on the bottom of your belly?

But if the client's words are so far removed from any you know, check that you really understand what he's referring to. If he mentions his 'waterworks', is he talking about his bladder or his tear ducts? Similarly, it's good practice to make sure that he's understood what you've been saying. This is particularly important when making the initial contract. The principle of informed consent requires that the client has been given all the relevant information, has indicated that he understands it and agrees to your terms and suggestions for treatment.

Blocks to communication

While it is important to listen well and to express ourselves as articulately as possible, there are certain ways of saying things which can hinder or facilitate communication between us and our clients. One of my clients said that she would like it better if she didn't feel silly every time she left the hospital. No one likes to feel belittled. There are some ways of speaking that are best avoided because they constitute major blocks to good communication.

Criticism, judgement and moralising

Of course, complementary therapists don't do any of these things with our clients. Or do we? One of the things that I've learned from clients is that what seems like an innocent observation to me can, by some people, be perceived as a criticism. If I tell Katy that her shoulder muscles are rather tight this week, she takes my comment to mean that I know she hasn't been doing her relaxation exercises and I'm telling her off. So I preface my observation with 'This isn't a criticism, but I've noticed that...'.

Because our business is to help people towards healthier ways of being, part of our work is to evaluate a client's lifestyle. Depending what sort of therapy we practise, we might ask about diet, sleep patterns, alcohol intake, past traumas, exercise routines, occupation or current relationships, in order to understand the client, and her problems, in the wider context of her life. Sometimes the responses to our questions may deviate considerably from what we might consider normal, acceptable, healthy or desirable. It's difficult not to feel critical of someone who says 'I spend about two hundred pounds a week on alcohol' or 'I don't need to exercise, I vacuum the carpet every day' or 'I eat three bars of chocolate for my lunch.' At which point comments about damage to health or irresponsible behaviours aren't helpful. Even a raised eyebrow or muttered 'Tut tut' could be construed as judgement.

Suppose for one moment that you are a smoker with a 40-a-day habit, a chronic nasty cough and a terror that you have lung cancer. You've tried everything you can to quit. A friend recommends a CAM practitioner. You tell her about the smoking and your attempts to stop. Which of these responses might encourage you to go further and confide your fears about cancer?

- I can understand why you'd want to stop. That's a nasty cough you've got there.

- You do know that your smoking is a serious threat to your health?

- I could refer you to a stop smoking clinic.

- You're telling me you want to stop but nothing you try works.

- It does take a lot of willpower and discipline to stop smoking.

Only the fourth response is an observation free of any evaluation or criticism. The third one offers advice but implies that the practitioner can't help. The last one implies, indirectly, that the smoker hasn't got any willpower or discipline.

EVALUATING

When we are looking for connections that tie into our theories or thinking about what the person is saying, our attention is split and we are not with them in what they are telling us, we are looking at them. The key ingredient in an empathetic response is presence. Of course, as professionals we do need to evaluate the symptoms as they are presented to us, to diagnose, guess, intuit what is going on, relate the facts to our theories, come up with a plan of treatment options and offer them to the client. But first we have to listen.

ACTING DEFENSIVELY

If we are able to refrain from acting defensively when a client criticises us, then communication is more likely to be smooth and effective. While it is a natural response to want to deny allegations if they're untrue, or to defend our position, particularly if we're right (which, of course, we always are!), such strategies don't help a client to feel understood. If we can listen, repeat what we understand the client to be saying to us, maybe commenting on her emotional response as well, then she is more able to hear our side of the story. If it really is important.

Suppose you have a treatment from a chiropractor for a bad back, and afterwards the condition worsens for a few days. When you go for your next session you mention this and say that you wish he'd warned you that that might happen. Which of the following responses would you like to hear?

- But I did tell you. You can't have listened.

- I thought everybody knew that.

- Yes, I should've mentioned it. I'm sorry.

- I can't imagine why it got worse. Did you rest like I suggested?

Useful strategies for good communication

Just as there are some ways of saying things to be avoided, if possible, there are also strategies that make for good communication.

Mirroring

Repeating the key elements of what you have just been told shows that you have listened and understood and lets the speaker hear for himself what he's just said and encourages him to continue.

CLIENT: I went to the seaside at the weekend and the air seemed much better than here in the city. I could breathe more easily. I didn't have any of my coughing fits.

PRACTITIONER: The sea air helped your breathing.

CLIENT: Yes and because I wasn't coughing I slept better too.

Implication

Making a suggestion embedded in a sentence as if it's taken for granted that the other person will comply.

For example, 'When are you going to start exercising?' Implication: you are going to start exercising.

'If you bend your knees, your lower back will feel more comfortable.' Implication: you will bend your knees.

'When will you be able to see your doctor?' Implication: you are going to see your doctor.

Positive questioning

Asking closed questions that require a 'yes' answer at the beginning of a case history facilitates a good working alliance. Your name is Mrs Smith? And your doctor referred you to me? You want to get rid of your headache as soon as possible?

Reframing

This means what it says: literally, taking a view of the world, a picture, and presenting it in a new frame. Same picture, same view, but looking different. The viewer might notice details that had been obscured in the old frame, certain features might seem brighter or fade into insignificance. When applied to a point of view, reframing means offering an alternative way of seeing or understanding without implying that the original is faulty or wrong.

In my grandfather's house, when I was a child, a portrait in a large ornate frame hung at the end of a dark corridor. The face scared me, because the eyes followed me as I walked towards then away from the painting. When my grandfather moved house, the portrait was cleaned and hung in the airy hallway. The man was frightening no longer; his eyes, in this new light, seemed sad and anxious instead.

I recall telling a friend the story of my birth by Caesarean section, with my mother and my baby self as traumatised victims and the operating surgeon cast as the villain. 'He was doing his best to make sure you were born alive', she said simply, reframing in a moment the view I'd held for many years of my difficult entry into the world.

Reframing sentences begin tentatively, offering an alternative interpretation, rather than proclaiming it loudly. They could begin with such phrases as:

- 'I wonder if…'
- 'Have you ever considered…'
- 'Then again, I suppose it's always possible that…'

To the client who is complaining that her body is letting her down by getting sick when she has so much to do – so many deadlines, committee meetings, parent teacher governor duties – a suggestion that maybe her body is indicating that she needs a rest is a reframing statement.

Respect

We demonstrate respect by accepting the client's frame of reference even if it seems very strange. Jeanette was a middle-aged woman who had been brought up in a fundamentalist religion, and although she had lost her faith, when she discovered she had breast cancer, she genuinely believed that the disease was God's punishment for giving her baby up for adoption when she was 20.

Authenticity doesn't require you to agree or accept the client's view point but accept that it is her way of seeing the world and if you can see if from that perspective too, communication will be enhanced.

Respect for other frames of reference is also important. Lower back pain could be understood to be:

- degeneration of the lumbar-sacral disc

- tension in the gluteal muscles

- a problem with grounding, poor contact with earth energy

- holding in the pelvis caused by too early toilet training

- imbalance in the kidney meridian.

Whichever framework you use, respect others. As Buddhists say, honour all traditions. None of the above is more 'true' than another. Some clients may come to us with complaints and dissatisfaction about traditional medical practice and it's important that we don't collude with running down doctors and the medical profession. It's unprofessional for a start and, in an environment that is attempting to be accepting and allowing, adds a jarring note.

Allowing the client to communicate clearly

The power imbalance in the relationship means that a conversation between a CAM practitioner and a client isn't balanced like a conversation between friends, with each party feeling that she has equal right to speak, disagree, butt in, change the subject or stop listening. During recent news programmes about the proliferation of superbugs in hospitals caused by poor standards of hygiene, patients on the wards who were told to complain if nursing staff didn't wash their hands, or the rooms weren't cleaned, replied that it wouldn't be in their best interests, and they might suffer poor treatment, or be labelled as a 'difficult patient' as a result. Even though many CAM clients pay for their treatments and have the power to change practitioner if they are not satisfied, it can still be hard to be assertive in the patient/client role.

We need to be mindful of this, particularly those practitioners who offer relaxation or general healing therapies rather than therapies that diagnose and cure. Some therapies are practitioner led; the client brings her problems and concerns and the practitioner makes suggestions for treatment and aftercare. This would be the case for acupuncture, chiropractic, medical herbalism, homeopathy, aromatherapy or reflexology. Others involve more negotiation between practitioner and client. During a massage, for example, the practitioner asks her client about pressure and speed of strokes and general comfort. In my experience, during an initial session very few clients dare to ask for something other than what I'm offering.

Non-violent communication

Non-violent, or compassionate, communication (NVC) is a process used around the world in homes, schools, workplaces and political situations. Marshall Rosenberg, a psychiatrist and mediator and creator of NVC, says: 'Non violent communication helps us connect with ourselves and each other in a way that allows our natural compassion to flourish. It fosters deep listening, respect and empathy and engenders a desire to give from the heart' (Rosenberg 2005).

NVC takes the values of unconditional positive regard, empathy, respect and authenticity, which are indispensable to good human relationships, and builds on them, creating a learning programme that is skills based. It teaches how to listen and speak without moralising, judging or using any of the blocks to communication mentioned earlier. There are four steps. These apply to the listening and the speaking part of the communication process. It doesn't matter if the other person isn't using NVC.

1. Observing what is happening, as it is, without evaluating it except in a basic way of 'is this OK for me' or 'not OK for me'? Do I like it or not?

2. Noticing how I am feeling as a response to what I am observing.

3. Becoming aware of the needs behind the feelings.

4. Formulating a request that will make my life better based on my observation, feelings and needs and that doesn't blame or criticise the other.

Here's an example.

Natalie didn't turn up for her session and didn't call until the following day to explain why she hadn't shown up. The underground train she'd been travelling on was stuck in the tunnel for half an hour, making her too late to come and preventing her from using her mobile to call me. At her next appointment I remind her that she would have to pay for the session she missed. 'But that's unfair!' she exploded. 'It wasn't my fault that I didn't get here. And I really wanted to come last week.' Once I might have said, 'I'm sorry but you know my cancellation policy. You do have to pay.' (Criticism: You've forgotten my policy. Moralising: You do have to, you must.)

Using NVC, I observe the following: Natalie is upset; she thinks I'm being unfair, she doesn't want to pay me and I don't much like any of this. I feel irritated, guilty and manipulated. My need is not that I have a rule and I don't like it being broken but that I want acknowledgement for the time that I was there, waiting for her. So instead I might say, 'You sound angry that I'm asking you to pay for the session that you missed, for something you didn't have through no fault of your own. I feel badly about charging you, but I was here for you for that hour last week and I need some acknowledgement of that.'

If you want to know more about NVC go to the website www.nonviolentcommunication.com.

The core conditions

Psychotherapists today generally agree that there are certain characteristics, often called the core conditions, that count a lot toward establishing a good working alliance with a client. Carl Rogers (1951), founder of Rogerian therapy, first proposed these over 50 years ago. Since there is quite a lot of evidence to show that therapists who demonstrate these characteristics have a higher success rate, I think it's worth thinking about them.

The core conditions are:

- unconditional positive regard

- congruence or 'being real'

- empathy and respect.

Unconditional positive regard

Love is a tricky word to use in a therapeutic context. It's used almost exclusively in popular culture to mean falling in love, or as a synonym for sex, and all the other variants like maternal love, filial love, love for one's fellow human beings, or spiritual love have less of a place in common currency, so I guess it was easier for Carl Rogers to describe the feelings of a therapist for his or her client as unconditional positive regard than unconditional love. Unconditional positive regard is about acceptance, about taking someone as you find them, about seeing through the personality traits or the physical symptoms to the real person behind all that. Acceptance means treating the client as an equal and treating his thoughts and feelings with sincere respect, even if you don't agree with them yourself. It does not mean thinking or feeling the way he does or valuing what he values.

Sometimes it isn't easy to accept people who have totally different views from ours, or who behave in ways that we wouldn't. I think it helps, in these sorts of situations, to separate the person from his behaviour. A child who is rude is not a bad child; she's a child who's behaving badly. A client who's surly is not a bad person; he's a person who has probably got something going on for him which results in him behaving impolitely. A woman who's irritable is not a bad person; she's a woman affected by her premenstrual hormones. A client who's joined the British National Party is not a bad person; he's someone whose politics and beliefs I don't share, but I respect his right to hold those beliefs.

But this is also where boundaries come in. Unconditional positive regard does not mean accepting behaviour or attitudes within the therapeutic context that are not appropriate. For example, while I know that smoking carries health risks and isn't an activity that I condone, I also respect people's right to smoke. But not in my treatment room. That's my boundary. One of my supervisees, Jane, is often in trouble because she's let yet another client leave with a promise that she'll get her money later. 'I'm such a nice person,' she says. 'It never occurs to me that a client would rip me off. I trust everyone.' Jane doesn't want to believe that some people aren't trustworthy. This isn't unconditional positive regard, it's naivety and a boundary issue that Jane needs to learn to deal with firmly. Unconditional positive regard doesn't mean letting others walk all over us.

Some people are harder for us to accept and love than others. When I used to teach children with special needs, there were always some who I'd take to right away, who had endearing little habits, were affectionate or pliable or eager to please me. And there were the difficult ones, the ones with behaviour problems, the ones withdrawn into their own worlds and unreachable, and the aggressive ones who fought or bit. I had to work much harder to connect with these children, to find ways of entering their worlds because they certainly had no motivation to enter mine. I had to accept frustration and disappointment, but ultimately, if I persevered, the bonds that I formed with these difficult children were so much stronger than with the so-called easy ones. These children taught me such an invaluable lesson. Whenever I meet a new client I have faith that I'll be able to reach them on some level, that a connection is possible even though it might not seem like it at first. I also remember something that one of my fellow teachers said, a throwaway comment about the children but a real eye opener for me. 'We've all got the same souls,' she said. I guess that unconditional positive regard might mean holding in mind that we all have the same souls.

But we also need to have unconditional positive regard for ourselves and be able to accept that there may always be times – when we are feeling low, in need of a holiday, or generally exhausted – when it is hard to summon genuine acceptance for others. And there may always be some people who we find difficult to relate to. The exercise 'projections and individual clients' (page 148) will clarify who that might be! And in these instances the best thing is to remember that it is not a good thing to work with people you dislike or can't accept.

LOVING KINDNESS MEDITATION

This exercise is a Buddhist practice. The aim of the loving kindness meditation is to cultivate a sense of unconditional friendliness and warmth towards all beings, no matter who they are or what they've done, including yourself. Loving kindness is an altruistic practice that we do for the benefit of others rather than ourselves and it helps cultivate unconditional positive regard. It is human nature to have positive and negative thoughts and some people who come into our lives arouse more negative thoughts, usually accompanied by hostile feelings, than others. When we think negative, we feel negative. Loving kindness meditation is a way to keep our minds from going sour.

The practice

Sit quietly and let your mind settle. Next bring an image of yourself to mind, as if you're looking in a mirror. Imagine yourself smiling warmly. This may be hard – don't worry, keep practising. Send warm loving feelings from your heart centre to yourself or try saying 'May I be well and happy'.

Then imagine in front of you someone you love and respect, such as an older family member or a beloved teacher, or someone very dear to you, perhaps a child you know. It's probably not a good idea to use your lover for this practice, because loving kindness feelings can easily tip over into sexual feelings! Look at this person's face and imagine him or her smiling back at you. Send warm loving feelings or say 'May she or he be well and happy'.

Then do the same with a person you feel neutral about, a person who doesn't kindle any particular feelings in you, someone who works in a shop you visit, for example.

Next, imagine someone you are having problems with, someone you hate or are angry with or want to avoid. Try to ignore your difficult feelings and focus on sending warmth and love. Imagine him or her gazing at you with warmth and joy.

Finally, imagine your feelings of warmth and love, care and concern for well being spreading outward from yourself and the other three people in your meditation to encompass all people everywhere. Say 'May all people everywhere be well and happy'.

Congruence/being real/being authentic

The dictionary defines congruence as agreeing with or corresponding to. In the context of interpersonal skills, as I think Carl Rogers intended it to be meant, congruence doesn't mean agreeing with another person, but rather that your own thoughts, feelings and actions are congruent, or agree with each other. Have you ever said, 'I'm so glad you could make it' when someone you don't like much arrives for dinner, or 'Thank you so much, it's just what I wanted' on opening a truly unpleasant birthday gift? These examples might be white lies, necessary to oil social relations, but they are also examples of incongruence. These are occasions when your true thoughts and feelings are kept hidden and you behave as if you felt something else. The way I understand it is that congruence in a therapeutic context is about being real or authentic, within certain limits. The self you bring to the therapeutic relationship isn't the same self you'd take to visit your mother, or to have a coffee with a friend or to the shops. Being real with a client isn't about sharing your holiday photos or your opinions on last night's television or the developments in your love life. It certainly isn't about asking your client for help or advice. Unlike other relationships, the one you have with the client exists only in the here and now and (usually) doesn't extend beyond the treatment room, so your life outside isn't relevant. The session time belongs to your client, and his concerns, not yours. A little ordinary chat at the beginning of a session oils the wheels, of course, and helps put people at ease but too much detracts from the real reason you're both there.

On a more subtle level, being authentic with the client in the here and now does involve your thoughts and feelings about him and the way you interact. It does mean responding genuinely to clients' stories or behaviour but with some discrimination. Thoughts about a person's appearance may be helpful (you look a lot better today than last time I saw you) or totally inappropriate (you look so silly in that woolly hat). I was once asked by a client if she looked all right with her hair coloured a particular way. I didn't want to give her my opinion, which was that I considered her pink hair at odds with her professional suits, so I suggested that perhaps she wasn't too comfortable with it, if she needed to ask my advice. Fortunately I found a way to be authentic without being hurtful. Usually I try to put my personal beliefs, tastes, values and experience on one side unless they are relevant to the situation and helpful to the client.

Empathy

> You can't know another man until you have walked a mile in his moccasins.
> (Native American saying)

Carl Rogers described empathy as being able to walk around inside another's world without ever losing a sense of your own self. Empathy is the ability to feel with another person and imagine what that person's life might feel like from the inside. There are various ways that you can gain understanding about a client. When you read a report about her from another professional the understanding you have is remote, from another source. When she tells you her story in her own words you can understand it using your own experience and identifying with her. The source you are using to understand her is your own self. Or you can attempt to understand alongside her, by 'putting yourself in her shoes'. This is empathy, the ability to understand 'as if' you are the other person.

Empathy isn't the same as sympathy, which is a particular feeling for or about another person, whereas empathy is feeling the feelings of the other person. We convey our sympathy for someone who has been bereaved, meaning that we feel sorry for him or her in the time of loss but we don't try and imagine what that person might be feeling. Of course, if we too have recently lost someone there might be a resonance, or identification – we can guess what he or she might be going through because it reflects our own experience.

The ability to be completely absorbed in a novel, a film or a play is a form of empathy. We 'lose ourselves' in the experience. But it's important not to lose ourselves in a client's world. What good can we be to anyone if we are lost? Successful empathy in the therapeutic relationship requires the ability to enter the client's world, but without losing our own sense of self. It's like listening to two stories at the same time; the one that the client is telling and the one that you are telling yourself. We listen to the words, the emotion behind them, body language, facial expression and we listen to our own body's messages, our own feelings. We learn to listen 'as if' we are the other person while at the same time listening in to our self.

TYPES OF EMPATHY

How we empathise depends a bit on our preferred mode of experiencing. We're trained to use our minds to understand things, so it's natural that we'll think about a person's experience and imagine what it might be like.

But empathy can occur without us being aware of it. Meeting a friend and sensing, even before she speaks, that something is wrong, walking into a room where a dispute is in progress and feeling the tension, or finishing a session with a client and feeling very sad, for no reason that you can think of, these are all examples of emotional empathy. Anxiety is a particularly contagious sensation too; stand in a queue in front of an anxious person and you can almost feel their adrenaline bombarding your body.

Twenty years ago it was common to hear healers and body workers talk about the importance of using protections or shields to avoid picking up 'negative energy' from clients. I was taught to surround myself with white light or to put cuffs of light around my wrist to prevent contamination. I was a bit sceptical, wondering what the fuss about a bit of negative energy was about, but more importantly, recognising that if I were to shield myself in that way, I'd also be screening out other information from the client and her body, which might be helpful in the work we were doing. I suspect that underlying these fears was the light/dark splitting that I discuss in Chapter 5 on power in the therapeutic relationship. And as my teacher, Jessica Macbeth, used to say when teaching in London from 1987 to 1989, 'Energy is only energy. How we interpret it depends on us. Feel it and let it go.'

Kinaesthetic empathy is the ability to feel what's going on in another's joints and muscles. It's also very easy, and, in fact, we all do it all the time when we mirror another's posture or gait or facial expression. I've heard at least two body therapists tell stories of learning about muscle action by copying the gait of people in the street and figuring out how they were using their muscles by paying attention to how it felt in their own bodies. Next time you have a drink with a friend watch how you both use your bodies; if you lean forward what does the other do? When you sit back, or lean on an elbow, watch your friend's response. One factor that may account for this unconscious mirroring is mirror neurons. Babette Rothschild (2006) describes how scientists have discovered the presence of certain visual motor neurons in the brain called mirror neurons. These neurons fire when you make a certain gesture, like picking up a cup. But apparently they also fire if you watch another person picking up a cup!

But how do we know what someone is feeling, on an emotional level? All emotions have an observable pattern of muscular responses, which are not culturally dependent. So, photos of people from Bali, China or Sweden who are happy all show the same facial characteristics, with the sides of the mouth raised and the eyes slightly opened. People from Pakistan, Iceland or Ireland who are feeling disgust will have wrinkled noses and tight throats. As we've already discussed, we have a tendency to copy other people's bodies. If we see a smiling face, we tend to smile. Now, every emotion also has a corresponding pattern of invisible bodily responses, governed by the autonomic nervous system, and involving breathing, heart rate, blood flow and sympathetic/parasympathetic predominance. For example, joy, fear, anger and excitement are sympathetic emotions while shame, sadness and peace are parasympathetic emotions.

To prove the point, try this little experiment. Come into your body and breathe. Then smile. It doesn't matter if there's anything to smile about or not. Notice what happens to your inner sensations when you move the muscle around your mouth into a smile. Stop smiling, let the edges of your mouth turn down, and slouch. Let your spine curve and your shoulders hunch forward. What happens to your inner sensations? How do you feel now? Just adopting the muscular patterns associated with an emotional response triggers that feeling.

Exercise to explore your communication style
Read the following, as if someone were actually talking to you and then read the responses. Which one would you most likely use?

Example one
You know, when I was in that training group, there was one person who really got to me. Most of the other students I liked, and the teacher was very good too. But this woman, well, I just couldn't stand her. She always sat in the front, and talked loudly, had an opinion on everything, been there, done that, what she was doing in the class I don't know, bloody know it all. Excuse my language, but she made me just mad. It got so that every time she opened her mouth I wanted to scream. I can't stand people who think they're better than others.
Responses:

  1. Oh yes, that reminds me of the girl I used to sit next to at school, very clever, and let me know it.

  2. Don't let people like that bother you, it's not worth it.

  3. Why didn't you complain to the teacher?

  4. You sound really agitated. I wonder what exactly it was about her that got to you?

Example two (from an elderly woman)
These young girls, when I see them on the street, wearing next to nothing, skirts up to their bums, bellies hanging out, jumpers so tight you can see it all, then I think, well they must be freezing in this weather, why don't their mothers make them dress properly? My mum would have never have let me out like that. And then, I think too, they're asking for it, how do they expect men to treat them with respect, dressed like that. So inconsiderate too. When I get on the bus, they all push me and act like they own the world, shouting and talking on their mobiles all the time.

Responses:

1. Yes, when I was on the bus last week, I saw two young girls sitting in priority seats. And they didn't stand up when an elderly person, with a stick, got on.

2. Young people are all the same, you shouldn't worry about them.

3. You shouldn't let them treat you badly.

4. It's not easy getting older, is it?

Example three (from a post office worker)
I've been in the sorting office 20 years now, I'm just sticking it out to my retirement. Not many white faces left now. When I started it was all Londoners and Irish. Now it's all Nigerians and it's got so racist. The other day, my line manager was on my back. Five minutes late in and he made me sign the late book, then all shift he was at me, hurry up Steve, you're behind schedule, look at the clock. He's one of these blacks, but not African. Now, during the evening, Fred from the next station came in, he's a lazy so and so. He was talking to one of our workers for ten minutes, they're both African. My line manager was even harder on me then. Because I'm the white man and he's scared of the others. It's not right, it's not.
Responses:

1. My friend told me a similar story to that the other day.

2. Well, you were late, and maybe you weren't working fast enough. You must have deserved it.

3. You should file a complaint, go to personnel or something.

4. That must have seemed really unfair to you.

Which type of response would you feel most comfortable with? The first kind of response is an ordinary conversational device. It's like playing ball: the ball, or topic, is thrown by the speaker, picked up by the listener and thrown back. The second person adds an example from his experience, and the result is a mutual acknowledgement of a shared reality. This sort of dialogue gives both people a sense that they are in agreement, belong to the same sort of world, and, particularly if the topic is one of complaint, a joining together against 'them', the perpetrators of the problem. Ordinary conversational devices like this are not out of place in the relationship between CAM practitioner and client, because they put people at ease, but too much, particularly during a treatment, takes the focus away from the here and now, and can blur the boundaries between the professional and a friendship relationship.

The second kind of response, the kind that communicates that the speaker is making a bit of a fuss about nothing, isn't usually very helpful in a therapeutic context. It minimises the speaker's experience or beliefs, and can make a person feel a bit stupid. In some circumstances it can be useful if the aim is to normalise someone's experience. Often our clients' concerns can be alleviated if we can put them in context by explaining that their response, symptoms, whatever, are normal, and many people would experience the same. For example when Angela asked me if the funny sort of feeling she got in her tummy just before she went to the toilet meant there was something wrong with her I didn't tell her not to be daft. I questioned her a bit, found out more about the sensations and concluded she was describing the ordinary sensation of needing to defecate. Asking this question was a really good sign because it meant that Angela was beginning to inhabit her body properly, and this awareness, something we all take for granted, was a big breakthrough.

The third type of response gives advice. We give clients advice all the time; it's part of our job. Depending on our therapy, we advise on diet, exercise, stretches, supplements, rest and so forth. We advise clients to try other therapies, or to see their doctor. It would be unprofessional not to give advice. And, it's also helpful to ask ourselves the following questions: is the advice relevant to the client and his issues? Is it within our professional remit? Is it based on sound principles or merely what I believe in? And, maybe most important, is it advice that this person needs right now, or does she just need me to listen? As good carers, we like passing on our wisdom, and giving clients tips and suggestions is another way in which we help them get better. It makes us feel good too. When Celia, a regular massage client, came in with bad pain, one side, lower back, and I was able, after treating her and after discussing what she'd been doing that might have caused the difficulty, to pinpoint it to picking up and putting on a heavy rucksack, she was impressed, and I felt pretty pleased with myself too.

But there are occasions, for all of us, I suspect, when we give advice because we can't think what else to do, because we can't bear someone's suffering, or don't really want to listen to what they're saying. This is where the fourth response is helpful. This type doesn't address the content of the speaker's communication, and it doesn't carry any of the listener's response either. What it does is address the speaker's feelings, either those that are being expressed in the here and now, as in 'you sound quite upset', or those that the listener guesses the speaker might have felt at the time, as in 'I imagine you felt quite angry/irritated/proud when that happened'. This is a really useful tool, for several reasons. The listener feels heard, and may feel encouraged to say more. The speaker can respond without having to comment on the content of the speech, a particularly useful ploy if you don't agree with what the speaker is talking about. It empathises with the speaker's feelings, which are body orientated, rather than her thoughts, which are mind orientated, taking the focus out of the head into the body, which is the domain of complementary therapy.

Exercise to practise empathetic responses

Compose a response to each of the following statements that addresses the feelings that are being communicated.

1. I'm sorry I'm late, the buses were terrible and I didn't know how far this place was and I got off at the wrong stop.

2. Can I show you a photo of my son? Here he is, he just finished his degree.

3. I don't think this knee is ever going to get better now. The operation didn't work.

4. When I went to my slimming club, I'd lost four pounds last week!

5. Since I lost my husband, I've no energy at all. Some days I could stay in bed all day.

6. Those doctors at the hospital are useless, I see a different one each time, have to wait hours, and then they've lost my notes!

7. I'm 80 next month, you know. And I swim every day, and do a yoga class.

8. I really thought that last remedy was the one. My rash began to clear, but then it came back, as bad as ever.

When the core conditions aren't in place…

In theory it's easy to agree that unconditional positive regard, empathy and respect are good qualities to cultivate towards the people we work with, and that communication is easier if we are real rather than coming from some false professional self, but it's also true that as human beings we're not always full of love and light and there are always going to be some people that we find it difficult to like. How do we accept these ones, who rub us up the wrong way or push our buttons? This is where some understanding of psychotherapy comes in useful. Psychotherapeutic wisdom would suggest:

- No one can make you feel anything. You are responsible for your feelings, although other people, or the things they say or do, might act as triggers.

- What projections are going on here?

- Is there a transference–countertransference dynamic being enacted?

Projections and transference are discussed in detail in Chapter 8 on psychotherapy terms.

The first thing to understand is that as the practitioner it's your responsibility to try to figure out what might be happening in the relationship. This includes your own feelings and attitude to clients. It isn't the client's job to behave better (unless she is breaking boundaries) or to be a nicer person or to stop reminding you of your older brother. The client is just fine as she is – it's you who's having the difficulty. The next is to decide if you really want to invest time and energy figuring out what's going on. Remember, you'll learn more about yourself than the client, and whatever happens, the situation between you and the client will change. The following exercises are tools for you to use on your own, to be your own supervisor, if you like, or a detective looking for clues to solve a mystery. These are not things to discuss with your client.

✍ Exercise to explore general difficulties with clients

It may be that there are certain client groups or characteristics that are hard for you to relate to easily. Have writing materials available, and make sure you won't be interrupted.

1. Make a list of all the clients you've ever worked with that you've found difficult. At this stage it doesn't matter why. Do it without thinking.

2. Next to each one write the reasons why you found them difficult, something about how they behaved, their attitudes, mannerisms, or how you feel with or after seeing them.

3. Look at your list again. Is a pattern beginning to emerge?

✍ Talking to your client as if...

This exercise comes from Gestalt therapy and is called a two chair exercise. Read through the whole exercise first then allow yourself enough time and privacy to do it properly. You need two chairs or cushions and writing materials.

Sit opposite an empty chair or cushion and imagine the person you are having difficulties with sitting there, bringing them to mind as clearly as you can. Then imagine what you would like to say to him as if he was really there and as if you weren't really a careful responsible practitioner. You can say anything you like – what you think of the person, how you feel when with them, what it is you can't stand about them, and so on. It's more effective to speak out loud but if you feel embarrassed you can say what you think in your head. Continue until you've finished.

Now for the hard bit. Switch chairs. Go and sit on your 'client's' chair. Look over at the 'practitioner's' chair and bring to mind as much as you can remember of what has just been said. You won't recall it all, don't worry. Notice what it's like to sit on this side, and how you are in your body and your feelings.

Return to your original chair and, if you like, make notes of what you discovered. Then think about the following questions:

1. How do you feel about your client now? At times, just venting can be enough to shift feelings.

2. Is there anyone that your client reminds you of? It may be that the strength of your reaction to this person lies in the way she reminds you of someone with whom you have or have had a strong emotional tie. If this is the case, look again at your client on the chair and say very clearly that you know your client is not your mother/last head teacher/Mrs Thatcher, that she is Mrs Brown, or Joan or whatever her name is. If this sounds too easy or a bit silly, it is both – but it can work!

At the end of this exercise, it's good practice to destroy written material or delete it from your computer, just in case anyone should take it for case notes.

Using focusing as a tool to explore a difficulty with a client

Another way to explore what's going on, particularly if you experience the difficulty in a diffuse way that's hard to get a handle on, is to use focusing. This was described in Chapter 2 on self care and resources. It's a good exercise for those who find it easy to relate to internal sensation.

1. Sit quietly and comfortably and let yourself settle.
2. Bring your 'difficult' client to mind, imagine what he or she looks like, and remember the last session.
3. Now turn your attention inwards, to your own body. What's going on? Scan your body and notice if there's a particular area or sensation that is calling your attention to it.
4. Focus on this sensation and wait. Don't try and think about it or what it means, just be with it. Wait for thoughts or other sensations or emotions to arise.
5. Maintain a patient-interested curiosity to your inner sensations. Allow them to speak to you. Ask them what they mean – be careful not to let your head get in there and decide for them!

Using imagery as a tool to explore a difficulty with a client

If you visualise easily, this is a good exercise for you.

1. Sit quietly and comfortably and let yourself settle.
2. Imagine you are sitting in a little film studio, just you and a projector. Or sitting facing your computer screen.
3. Bring your 'difficult' client to mind, imagine what he or she looks like, and remember the last session.
4. Then ask for an image of your client to be shown on the screen.
5. Wait. Just allow whatever emerges. What's your reaction to this image? Do you like it? Does it make any sense to you? Does it help you understand your client or what's going on any better?

If the image isn't particularly helpful, sit with it for a while to see if any insights occur at a later moment.

Examples of using these exercises

Carl is a massage client. I'm finding that I'm not looking forward to seeing him and wonder why, so I try the two chair exercise. This is what I find myself saying.

Before you come, when I see your name in my appointment book, my heart sinks, I really don't want you to come, I hope you'll cancel. It's almost dread, this sinking feeling. And yet I know when you walk in, with your little smile and your 'how are you?', which sounds genuine, then I'll be pleased to see you. It isn't about your big body or your clumsiness, they don't bother me even though I know I'd think you a bit odd if I saw you on the street, a stranger. I want to say to you don't come, go away, I don't want you. But I could never say that to your sweet innocent face; it would be so hurtful. And then I switch to the other chair and, as 'Carl', feel horribly hurt and rejected as I remember what's been said. At this point I remember that he has told me, in passing, about being bullied at school. I begin to wonder whether this man is communicating his concern that I might reject him too. Outside the session, before he arrives, I'm behaving like others have in his past. As if I too am a rejecting person. I'm certainly having those sorts of feelings. I leave it there, feeling that I now have a way of understanding my own reactions. And guess what? I never find myself dreading his appearance again. Whether I was correct in my assessment or not doesn't really matter. The point was that I was no longer puzzled by my own reactions.

Katie is a psychotherapy client. She has issues with her weight. I work too hard with her and sometimes feel scrutinised and generally uncomfortable. I used the imagery exercise to explore this. Here's what happened: first I saw a big toad squatting on my sofa, looking at me with big watery bulgy eyes, as if it was trying to eat me up or get inside me. No wonder I felt uncomfortable. Then I looked again and for a while nothing came. I was looking at a blank screen. Then something caught my eye, in the bottom left-hand corner of the screen. It was a very small image of a dumpy toddler holding out her arms to me...and when I understood that the blown-up toad image was a front for an insecure child my attitude softened. I keep this image in mind whenever Katie is being her most obnoxious.

5

Power in the Therapeutic Relationship

Power as a negative concept

The idea of power holds negative connotations for many of us. Notice your own reactions to this statement: 'As a complementary therapist/practitioner I have more power than my client.'

When a group of massage therapists who'd met to explore the notion of power in the therapeutic relationship read this sentence there was a collective gasp, followed by comments ranging from 'dream on...what an outrageous statement!' and 'I hope not. That statement takes me out of the therapeutic relationship to any other place' to 'I disagree. Anyone who says that is more interested in themselves than in the client.' There was a strong feeling in the group that the practitioner was certainly not more powerful than the client, and that the relationship was, or should aim to be, a mutual one, with power, and responsibility for the outcome of treatment, shared between practitioner and client.

Mitchell and Cormack, in their book *The Therapeutic Relationship in Complementary Health Care* (1998), also describe how practitioners can feel uncomfortable with the notion of a power imbalance.

> On the one hand, the desire to be liked by one's patients and to be seen as warm, caring and compassionate can lead to a pretence that there is little or no difference between the patient and practitioner...on the other hand...power may be so taken for granted that they do not realise they have it. (p.91)

Power as a neutral force

Where do we get the idea that power is a bad thing? When the group tried to define power, the words strength, abuse of power, overruling, struggle, politics, government, greed, competition, potent, control and misuse of power came up, most of which refer to power as a force for control and domination. In Collins English Dictionary (1998) there are 20 different definitions of the word power. Here are the first four:

1. ability or capacity to do something

2. a specific ability, capacity or faculty

3. political, financial or social influence

4. control or domination or a position of control or domination.

The first three in this list refer to power as an ability or a capacity to do or to influence something. Of itself, power is a neutral force. It's how the force is expressed and how it is used that makes the difference. Consider energy, emotion and touch. Like power, these are also neutral forces. A touch can be healing or abusive depending on the intention of the giver, the force with which it is given, and the context in which it occurs. A hard slap on the back could save someone's life if he is choking but feel very different if it happened during a domestic argument. Energy can be enlivening or sapping, calm or jittery, smooth or jagged. An explosion of rage has destructive potential, but we talk about having a 'good' cry. Power exists on a continuum, with positive use at one end, the notion of power as an enabling, facilitative force for change and negative at the other, with power used as a dominating, controlling and suppressive force.

Maybe this story will help to illustrate the notion of power as a neutral force.

Two people, an elderly woman and a young man, are travelling on foot along a road. The man falls and twists his ankle. Unable to stand up, he reaches out his hand to the woman who has a choice. She can give assistance or she can walk away. At that moment, where one is vulnerable and the other is not, the person who is on her feet and who can offer help is the more powerful. At that moment, she could use her relative health and strength to help the man up, in which case she'd be using her power as a force for good. But if she laughed, kicked the man and walked away, she'd be choosing to use her relative power in a destructive way.

In many other circumstances, the woman would be considered less powerful than the young man. She'd probably not be as strong physically, might have less income, and as a woman and an elder she has less social status. Power is not only a neutral force, but also a relative one. When our clients come to us they, like the young man in the story, are vulnerable and need a helping hand. They come with the expectation that we will extend our hand in return, not that we will kick them. When a client walks through the door, we, like the elderly woman, are in a position of relative power. We have chosen, by virtue of being complementary therapists, to help others and with that decision comes power, not in the sense that the word is often understood, but in the sense that we are in a position to facilitate healing.

We have earned the power that enables us to help. We are the ones with the diplomas, certificates, skills and experience and all of this entitles us – and our clients – to believe that we have the means to help them. The movement towards standardisation of training and registration of practitioners within complementary therapy reflects our professionalism and ensures the public that we are not sham practitioners, that we are not quacks. In this respect we are not equal (unless we are treating another therapist) and I think most clients would be horrified if we pretended not to know any more than they did. Clients are experts in their own bodies, because, after all, they've lived in them for years and know how they feel, what they like and dislike, but that doesn't mean that our clients know all about acupuncture meridians, homeopathic remedies or deep tissue release – that's why they've chosen to consult one of us. And in recognition of this difference, there's usually a financial contract, whereby the client pays the practitioner for services rendered (or the clinic, or, if the service is being provided within the NHS, pays indirectly through taxes and national insurance contributions).

As a practitioner, I have a responsibility to myself and my clients to be in good shape, physically, mentally and emotionally. If I'm not, I need to consider taking time out from work to look after myself. In this respect, I should be in better health than my clients. When a client walks through the door, he has an unspoken assumption that the practitioner is fit to work with him. Here is another, relative, power imbalance; one person is in a better state of health than the other.

Here we tread a fine line between self care and the assumption that we, the healers, are well and they, the clients, are sick. This power imbalance is completely relative. I can only be a good healer to the extent that I know my limitations, my weaknesses and my own potential to be sick.

Power and touch

Many complementary therapies require that the client lies down, and some also ask that she remove some or all of her clothes. There is an unspoken assumption on both sides that the practitioner may touch the client, but not the other way round. It isn't hard to see that the person who is supine, naked and prepared to be touched is more vulnerable and therefore less powerful than the person who is clothed, standing and doing the touching. There are many studies of social status and touch and, without being consciously aware of it, we abide by the rules regarding touch of the culture we were brought up in. If you are a white English man from a tough inner city area then physical contact with male relatives and friends will be minimal, especially in public, but if you are from a Mediterranean country you will consider it quite ordinary to hug, kiss or walk arm in arm with your male friends in the street. And all over the world adults pat, stroke, tickle and pick up small children whether they want to be touched or not. Children, the very elderly and the very sick have little power to determine the type or intensity of touch they receive. Some cultures touch a lot more than others, with Britain and North America among the least touching countries.

Underlying reasons for our discomfort

But even if we can acknowledge the power that our qualifications, relative health, our place on a register, our years of clinical experience and the imbalance in the therapeutic relationship as a result of this, we may still feel uncomfortable with this idea of power.

Let's consider the underlying reasons for this. On the one hand we are not doctors in white coats, or the stereotypical aloof consultant or a general practitioner who prefers the sight of the computer screen to the sight of a patient. We are not the sort of professionals who claim to know best, whose authority mustn't be questioned, who expect our patients to cooperate with our given treatment without question. Of course this description is exaggerated and unfair to all those who have trained and work in allopathic medicine, but there is some truth in the belief that conventional medicine looks at the symptoms first and the person second, and that complementary therapies try to do the opposite, and, moreover, encourage active patient/client participation in the healing process. The way that power is used in traditional medicine can seem controlling or dominating, not a model that complementary therapists condone.

Another source of discomfort lies in the connection between complementary therapy and the New Age movement. Although some therapies are far older than Western allopathic medicine, acupuncture and Ayurvedic medicine being good examples, many are less than a hundred years old, reflexology and craniosacral therapy being two examples in this category. The whole complementary therapy field has developed alongside an expansion of interest in meditation, Eastern religions, altered states of consciousness, past life experiences, angels and near death experiences.

My old teacher, Jessica Macbeth (2002), used to say that healing has become synonymous with spirituality, or following a spiritual path, and that no matter what belief system a person follows, the influence of the Judaic–Christian tradition is very strong. The spiritual life is one of self sacrifice, caring for others, devotion, purity and lack of interest in material matters, all of which sit uneasily with the idea of power. Buddhists, too, talk about a 'mutual co-arising' within any encounter between two people, meaning that, no matter how big the difference between them, each has something to offer the other that can help growth and change.

But I believe that it is only when we can acknowledge our relative power in the therapeutic relationship, and the choices we make when acting in our power, that we are in a position to empower the people we work with. There can be no mutuality unless the practitioner owns her own power.

Power over and power within

This brings us to another way of thinking about power. We've explored the idea of power as a neutral force, which exists along a continuum with abuse at one end and empowerment at the other. This concept implies a power that is conferred from outside, that comes with status, experience, or money. For example, the person who wins the lottery suddenly has a much greater spending power. The person elected prime minister takes on particular political powers with the job. These are powers that come from outside. But what about power that comes from within? Consider the power in a seed that forces the shoot through the seed case. Consider the potential within a child to grow and develop.

Power within, or personal power, refers to potential, energy or force to create, live more fully, fulfil our purpose, and determine our life's path, move, and play. This sort of power is associated with the second chakra, the one situated in the belly, and depends upon a healthy root chakra, supplying strong earthed physical energy, and a clear connection with the higher chakra to manifest this power in the outer world. Personal power is related to self esteem, confidence, and being at ease in the world.

Think about people you know whom you'd describe as powerful. What are their attributes? What distinguishes them from other people? What was it that enabled Nelson Mandela to survive his years in prison without losing his commitment to the black South African cause and to emerge as a powerful leader?

✍ **An exercise to relate to personal power**
Sit quietly and centre yourself.

Remember a time when you have felt powerless. Bring the whole experience to mind as fully as you can – relive the incident. Notice how you felt, emotionally and in your body. Then let it go. Take a deep breath and imagine releasing the memory on the out breath. Next, think of a time when you felt powerful. It may take longer for your memory to come up with something – we tend to recall difficult events more easily than positive ones. Again, relive it as much as you can focusing on your felt senses. How do these experiences differ? Make a note of how your body felt in both situations.

When we did this exercise in the group, Jane said:

> In the situation where I felt powerful, the less my ego was involved, the more powerful I felt. I had nothing to lose, there was nothing at stake and the more engaged I could be with the other person and the subject matter. But in the situation when I felt powerless I felt panic, withdrawal and I got littler and littler and my body became a tight little knot.

Powerlessness is often associated with feeling small or childish, not surprisingly. When we were children we were powerless.

6

Touch in the Therapeutic Relationship

The importance of touch has been acknowledged for a very long time; around 50 BC Lucretius likened touch to a paved road leading straight to the human heart and mind. Today, organisations like The Touch Institute in Miami are carrying out research to back up Lucretius' claim. There is evidence that touch is a crucial factor in the physical and emotional development of babies, and in adults can improve immune functioning, lower stress hormones, reduce pain and alleviate depression (see www.miami.edu/touch-research). Complementary therapists who contact clients' bodies directly as part of their work take it for granted that touch is healing. There are many forms of physical contact that could occur within the context of the therapeutic relationship, even for those practitioners who practise a non-contact therapy such as homeopathy.

Social and cultural norms

Touch between practitioner and client during a session could be initiated by either party, with the exception of therapeutic touch as part of the treatment. A client wouldn't be the one to give the aromatherapy massage, but might tap the practitioner's shoulder to get her attention or pat her on the head or give her a hug. However, given the power imbalance in the relationship, it is more likely to be the practitioner who does most of the touching. In any dyad, the person perceived to be more powerful is more likely to initiate contact than the other. So, adults touch children, doctors touch patients, tutors touch students, men touch women – but these days concerns about touch and harassment or accusations of abuse may constrain many individuals from ordinary, spontaneous use of touch. Fathers report feeling uneasy about showing affection to their small daughters in public, bosses are apprehensive about physical contact with employees and male teachers take great care never to be left alone with female students. Social touch is hedged round with fears of approbation, so all the more reason for complementary practitioners to be conscious of and monitor and take responsibility for how we use it, or accept client-initiated touch.

As well as social norms, there are cultural ones regarding not only who can touch who, but how often and where. Hunter and Struve (1998) list research showing that certain groups, among them Mediterranean people, Latin Americans, Greeks, Turks and some African peoples, engage in frequent physical contact, whereas North Americans, Germans and English people do not. Japanese people experience much physical contact in public, but are very restricted as to who and how often they can touch at home.

Each one of us has our own relationship to touch, both in terms of how easy it is to touch others and to allow them to touch us. This depends on our cultural and social background, but also on our personal experience of touching and being touched throughout our life. It used to be said that the growth of massage and bodywork therapies during the 1960s and 1970s was simply a way for the babies from the 1940s, who were fed on schedule and not picked up when they cried, to get their needs for holding on demand met. The following two exercises are to help you clarify your own relationship to touch. They are both 'write and reflect' exercises.

Your personal history of touch

1. How were you touched as a baby? What stories have you been told about this time in your life, about what sort of baby you were? Have you seen your mother (significant adult) handling other babies?

2. Were your family physically close? Did you get hugged and kissed a lot, or hardly touched at all? Was touch used for punishment? Was touch used inappropriately?

3. What sort of touch have you had from doctors or nurses? Have you had operations, or spells in hospital? Have you suffered from skin disorders?

4. Have you had any accidents in your life that have affected your body? Broken bones, or road traffic accidents or falls?

5. What's your best sexual memory?

6. And your worst?

7. Who touches you now in your everyday life, and how?

8. How are you feeling now, after thinking about all these personal questions?

Touch with different kinds of people

How might you feel if any of these people touched you on the arm during a conversation? Use your internal OK and not-OK signals to help:

- a woman friend
- a child
- a doctor
- a gay man
- your supervisor
- a man friend
- a shop assistant
- a white person (if you identify as black)
- a lesbian
- a much older person
- a shop assistant
- a black person (if you identify as white)
- a stranger at a bus stop
- your teacher/tutor.

How likely would you be to touch any of these people on the arm during a conversation:

- a woman friend
- a child
- a doctor
- a gay man
- your supervisor
- a man friend
- a shop assistant
- a white person (if you identify as black)
- a lesbian
- a much older person
- a shop assistant
- a stranger at a bus stop
- your teacher/tutor
- a black person (if you identify as white).

The meaning communicated by touch

Another point to bear in mind is that, as with any sort of communicative exchange, the meaning intended by the giver cannot be assumed to be the meaning understood by the receiver. A colleague told me about this exchange; her client had been talking at length about the problems in his sexual relationship. Wanting to get his attention back to the session, she leant forward and touched his leg. 'Oh,' he said, 'are you making a pass at me?' Because his mind was on sex, he understood the contact, in that moment, as sexual. As soon as he saw the look on the practitioner's face, he realised his mistake. And an outsider may misinterpret the meaning of touch between two people. Anyone watching Fran, a mental health user, and myself shake hands at the beginning of a session would think we were being polite and a bit correct. In fact, as we both know, this contact helps Fran to remember that I am a real flesh-and-blood person and not a cardboard cut out.

Unethical touch

Let's now consider the different kinds of touch that could, potentially, occur in the therapeutic relationship. Edward W.L. Smith describes a taxonomy of different kinds of touch in psychotherapy (Smith, Clance and Imes 1998). To start with, there are two kinds of touch that are unethical, inappropriate and harmful to the client. These are sexual touch and violent or aggressive touch. Touch that carries sexual intention on the part of the practitioner, or is designed to arouse sexual response in the client for the practitioner's gratification, is taboo. One possible exception would be in certain types of bodywork session where the specific and negotiated goal might be to release blocked erotic energy for the client's own benefit, for use in private life, not for the practitioner's in the session. Slapping, hitting, pushing, punching or restraining a client are obviously unacceptable in the treatment room. If a client refuses to leave the room, or becomes violent and a danger to himself or the practitioner, the first step, if possible, is to get outside help, so there is a third party as witness to any forceful touch that might be needed, either to restrain or evict. The intention behind such touch should, ideally, be non-retaliatory.

Touch as part of the therapeutic technique

Many complementary therapies involve skilful and intentional touch: to shift stagnant energy, align vertebrae, to energise an organ, to soothe pain, to improve joint mobility. We assume that a client who chooses one of these therapies understands that touch is involved but this may not be the case. Some of the more unusual forms of bodywork are not household names. Most people will know about massage or osteopathy, but Rolfing, Hellerwork or Trager are not names in the public arena. A person could, conceivably, visit a practitioner of one of these therapies on a friend's recommendation, without knowing what is involved. If this sounds farfetched, a more likely scenario in which the client may not understand that he will be touched is if he is a child, has learning difficulties or mental health problems. The nature of the contact and the reason for it needs to be explained – as it should, indeed, in a first session with any client, as part of the contract. Client must be told about the nature of the touch, the intention and possible outcomes, including adverse effects, in order to give informed consent.

Touch and pain

At times certain complementary therapy treatments may cause some level of pain. Pain is an unpleasant response associated with actual or potential tissue damage, or the perception of such tissue damage. There is always a sensory and an emotional component. Perception of pain is subjective, varying from person to person. There is no clear or consistent correspondence between the experience of pain and tissue damage. People have been known to perform amazing tasks with broken limbs if their lives are in danger. There is extensive tissue damage, but no pain. This only kicks in once the person is safe. On the other hand, people with amputated limbs may report pain, twitching or itching in a non-existent leg, a phenomenon that shows sensation in the absence of tissue (Wall 1999).

Within the therapeutic relationship, the crucial issue regarding touch and pain (apart from the obvious one of how best can the therapy be used to alleviate pain) is communication. Many of our clients have pain or discomfort of some kind or they wouldn't be coming to see us, even those who use complementary therapies as a preventative measure, to maintain fitness levels, experience minor stress-related symptoms. How clearly can the client describe her pain? Apparently there are over 70 words for it. The more information you have, the better you can devise a treatment plan, and evaluate its success. Words for pain fall into three categories; those that refer to the sensation of the pain, like pounding, itchy, sharp, aching, burning; words that describe the effect of the pain on the subject, like sickening, tiring, relentless, punishing, distressing; and words that describe the intensity of the pain, like mild, unbearable, strong. So, a possible dialogue to ascertain the client's experience of pain might go something like this:

CLIENT: It's in my left shoulder, it hurts when I move it like this [demonstrates abduction].

PRACTITIONER: What sort of hurt is it? Sharp or aching or something else?

CLIENT: No, it's more like a burning. Only when I move my arm. When it's still it aches.

PRACTITIONER: And on a scale of one to ten, how bad is it, if one is minimal and ten is unbearable?

CLIENT: Today it's a seven.

PRACTITIONER: That sounds quite painful. How does it make you feel?

CLIENT: It upsets me, I almost feel like crying when I get that burning feeling.

If the client can communicate about pain to you, do you, the practitioner, tell her about the possibility that your touch might be painful, that some parts of the treatment might cause discomfort? Ideally during the initial consultation, as part of information given to the client to allow her to give informed consent for the treatment, a client should be told if contact might hurt (and, in the case of non-contact therapies, that treatment might initially exacerbate symptoms, or bring about a healing crisis). When I was new to complementary therapy, I don't ever remember a practitioner telling me that a treatment might be painful and yet I've had an excruciating shiatsu session after which I promised my legs never to take them near that therapy again (I have, and had a different experience), had acupuncture which left me with sore spinal muscles for three days afterwards and experienced the unpleasant shock of sudden neck manipulations by osteopaths. Did I fail to register if practitioners warned me of possible discomfort or did they assume that I knew?

I think it helps to forewarn, without frightening the client, that some contact during the treatment may be painful, but, as well, to communicate that the client has permission to stop painful touch during the treatment. As children we learn to submit when adults get soap in our eyes, rip plasters off, take us to the doctor for inoculations or the dentist for a filling. We accept that some things will hurt and learn that complaining won't get us anywhere. I think we take this attitude to all our health-care professionals when we grow up. Many therapeutic interventions work best when the physical body is relaxed, and a body that is in pain, or anticipating it, is not relaxed. I talk with clients about the difference between 'good' pain, like the sort experienced when a tight muscle is squeezed hard to release tension, and 'bad' pain, the sort that comes with warning signs that something is happening that isn't in the body's best interests. People intuitively seem to know the difference and find it helpful to be told they have a responsibility to prevent the second sort happening.

Other kinds of touch

As well as the taboo kinds of touch, and intentional therapeutic touch which is part of the negotiated contract, such as effleurage, feeling for a pressure point, laying on of hands or rotating a joint, there are other sorts of physical contact that can occur in any practitioner–client relationship including those that don't use touch like homeopathy or medical herbalism. Accidental touch, social touch and touch for comfort are all in this category. Before we consider these in depth, try exploring how much of this sort of touch you use with clients.

1. Do you touch your clients when greeting them? All clients or only certain ones? And how?

2. Do you touch clients during consultation? If yes, how?

3. If a client becomes distressed, do you touch him or her? If yes, how?

4. Do you touch clients when saying goodbye? All clients or only certain ones? And how?

5. Do you touch clients at other times?

6. Do your clients ever touch you?

Accidental touch

Accidental touch is not intentional, consciously, at any rate, neither is it therapeutic. Treading on a client's toe, bumping into him, or brushing against him possibly indicates that the practitioner is in the client's personal space without permission and this could be felt as invasive. Inadvertent touch can occur during a treatment; a light touch on the breast when covering them with a towel, an arm resting on the belly or pubic bone unbeknown to the practitioner. In everyday life outside the treatment room, the normal and immediate response would be to apologise – so too within the therapeutic context. The practitioner might spend a moment, privately, wondering about any possible unconscious meaning in the accident. Here's an example that June, a recently qualified aromatherapist, brought to supervision. A client had asked June not to touch her feet because they were extremely sensitive and yet on two subsequent occasions she 'forgot' and found herself automatically ending the treatment holding the client's feet. June didn't understand how she could be so thoughtless. When we explored further, it emerged that this client was quite critical and managed to convey the impression that she found June incompetent. She was 'touching a sensitive spot' for someone not long in practice. On realising this, June could see her accidental foot touching as an unconscious retaliation and never needed to do it again.

Social touch

Then there is social touch, the contact made between two people on meeting and again on parting, and, possibly, during their interaction. Here there's a lot of cultural variation: white British shake hands on meeting, Eskimos rub noses and Japanese bow. Even within cultural norms, there are individual variations in use of social touch. The therapeutic relationship isn't a social relationship, so what is appropriate in the way of social touch? And should it be practitioner or client led?

I tend to be extremely cautious myself about social, or any non-negotiated touch, because I know how easily it can be misinterpreted. I use my own internal not-OK signals to monitor my behaviour. Even now, as I write, I can bring people that I have worked with to mind, imagine touching them, and have an internal response letting me know if it would be a good idea or not. When I remember that any contact is a two-way event regardless of who initiates the touch, I wouldn't necessarily assume that my reaction means that the other person doesn't want me to touch them. It could be a countertransference reaction (see Chapter 8), an unconscious communication from them to me. It could also be my personal antipathy to their physical presence. Whatever the reason for my response, I'd avoid initiating social touch.

Also, there's something about a boundary between the space where touch, sometimes very intense, personal, evocative touch occurs, which is (usually) on my treatment couch, and the space where we are two separate individuals, me sitting in my chair and the client sitting in hers. When we sit like this, as two adults discussing what will happen, I may touch to ascertain the exact location of discomfort, say, but otherwise not. During the treatment, I may never know exactly who I am for the other person. I don't know what my touch represents.

If the client has experienced emotional release, or regressed to a childlike place, or slept, or been in a deep inner world, she needs time and physical separation from me, to come back to her adult here-and-now self. So once the treatment is over, I don't touch again, except maybe to demonstrate a technique for the client to practise: a muscle stretch, for example. This is technical rather than social touch.

When I think about exceptions to this, when I might use social touch, there are ending sessions with clients who I have come to know over a period of time and who have finished treatment or are moving away. Complementary therapy treatments tend to be open ended; even if a fixed number of sessions has been agreed, the client always has the option of returning at some point in the future. But, sometimes, we know we are saying goodbye. This was the case with Rebecca, who was returning to Australia after three years working in

London and travelling in Europe whenever she had a free moment. She'd seen me once a month for massage. To refuse her hug at the end would have been churlish. It also marked the end of our professional relationship.

There are times when I've been the recipient of unwanted touch. Once or twice young women, who usually worked in fashion or media, have come over and kissed me on both cheeks before leaving. I guess this is normal behaviour in their social milieu; maybe it's a way of showing gratitude and maybe ignorance of the 'rules' of the therapeutic encounter. I don't expect to be kissed at the end of a session, it's not in my idea of the 'rules' so I don't kiss back – and usually it doesn't happen again.

Occasionally I get asked for a hug, and again, I use my gut response, and the context, and what I know of the client. So, for example, if a person is distressed, miserable and I know she's going home to an empty house, it would be unkind of me to refuse. But on other occasions I might say no, on the grounds that it would be unprofessional, if I sense that there's a sexual element, or that boundaries are being pushed.

Touch for comfort

This brings us to the last kind of touch, which is always intentional and intended to be therapeutic, although it may not be experienced by the client as such: touch as a tool to comfort or soothe a person in distress. This can range from a light touch on a shoulder, arm or leg to a prolonged cuddle. While it's a normal response, reaching out to touch someone who's upset, there are considerations within the therapeutic relationship. Who is the comfort for? Sometimes, behind our desire to soothe another, there lurks our own inability to bear the crying, to witness the pain or just be with another person without having to make it better. It can be very hard to allow another person to feel their pain. It can seem callous, watching and not trying to fix it. But rushing in too soon, with comforting hugs or tissues, may communicate that you don't want the person to be crying in your treatment room – that, in fact, you want her to pull herself together, quickly. This just adds to any embarrassment or shame about the emotional release in the first place. So, when a client is distressed and you have an impulse to touch, ask yourself: who is this touch really for?

7

Sex and the Erotic in the Therapeutic Relationship

Consider the following vignettes:

I felt twitches in my vagina, pleasurable contractions. It was a sunny Sunday morning in spring, two years after I had stopped seeing Adam. I was chopping some fennel when he not so much entered my mind as tapped on my body, as he had done so many times during the course of a five year therapy. (From 'The Vampire Casanova' in Susie Orbach, *The Impossibility of Sex*, 1999, p.7)

They both entered the treatment room and sat down. As the initial consultation progressed, James became aware that the woman talking to him in a gentle, husky voice was very sexy. He noticed her breasts moving as she breathed and became quite aroused. At last he couldn't stop himself: 'Look' he said, 'I'm really embarrassed about this, but I find you very attractive.'

A healer tells me that if her client is an attractive man, she'll rub her pubic bone surreptitiously against the corner of the table, to increase her erotic pleasure in the situation.

Gary works as a massage practitioner in an organisation for gay men with HIV. His predecessor was sacked for unprofessional behaviour and Gary is very careful, therefore, to maintain clear boundaries. On one hot summer day, a client asks if he can be massaged without towels, and throughout he flirts and pays Gary outrageous compliments. Gary reacts professionally and appropriately but nonetheless finds himself in a sexually charged state. Halfway though the massage with his next client he realises that he is working in an extremely sensual way, as if he were massaging a lover, as a means to discharge the erotic energy from the previous encounter.

Notice your reactions to these vignettes. Are you shocked? If so, by the content of the stories, or by the mere fact that someone is admitting to having sexual responses within a professional context? Have you ever thought about the place of sex and the erotic in your work, or do you assume that, because it is forbidden, you have no need to think about it? This is certainly the stance that most of our codes of conduct endorse quite explicitly. This is from the Code of Ethics and Conduct of the Craniosacral Therapy Association:

> 3.3.1 Serious difficulties will occur if you abuse your professional position to pursue an emotional (in a personal sense) or sexual relationship with a client or their close relative: this is bound to disturb the crucial relationship between practitioner and client. It is your professional duty not only to avoid putting yourself in such a position, and to avoid any form of behaviour which might be misconstrued in this way.

And this from the Massage Training Institute Code of Ethics: '3.4 Practitioners must not engage in sexual activity with their client.'

Sex and the erotic do not belong in the therapeutic relationship. But, like power, maybe sex is there whether we like it or not, and if we can begin to think about it, we may be less at risk of stepping over the boundaries and behaving unethically. 'Your thoughts create your reality' is a phrase often used today. Does this mean that if complementary therapists think about sex in relation to their clients that there will be an outbreak of sexual behaviour in treatment rooms? I think not. In fact, I think the opposite is true, that when difficult or forbidden thoughts and feelings can be expressed, there is far less chance that the thoughts will be acted upon. Derek Jehu's research in 1994 on the incidence of sexual abuse of clients by psychotherapists, psychiatrists and social workers in the USA and the UK suggested that as many as 10 per cent of these professionals had sexual contact with clients and that the majority, but not all, of the people who had had sexual contact with health-care professionals suffered harm as a result. No comparable research has been done with complementary therapists, and awareness of abuse issues is higher than it was over ten years ago, so we can't assume that one in ten of our professional colleagues is behaving inappropriately, but neither can we assume that it doesn't happen, or that none of us could find ourselves having sexual thoughts or feelings during our work.

Sex and taboos

David Mann suggests, in his book *Psychotherapy: An Erotic Relationship* (1997), that taboos and prohibitions exist to prevent human beings acting out certain powerful impulses. The stronger the urge to do something, the stronger the taboo to prevent it. The universality of the incest taboo may be based on an unconscious recognition that mixing genes from the same pool can have disastrous results but it may also reflect the strength of sexual desire. At its most basic, sex is a very powerful biological drive, stimulated by the sight and scent of, and physical contact with, another human being. When people live in close physical proximity, as they do in the family, the conditions exist for sexual arousal. The incest taboo prohibits family members from acting on their biological sexual urges — or should. Unfortunately, many children do suffer because family members aren't constrained by the taboo.

The taboo against sexual relationships in the psychoanalytic world is well documented. Many of the early analysts, Freud included, had contact with their female patients of a sort that would be considered completely unethical today. Jung had an affair with a patient, and both Melanie Klein and Freud analysed their own children. Although Freud originally believed that analysts needed to engage with the erotic aspect of the patient, he came to recognise that he couldn't maintain professional neutrality when faced with his young female patients' intense love for him, and changed his mind. It has been suggested that psychoanalysts retreated out of sight of their patients, sitting in a chair behind the analytic couch, in order to feel safer from their patients' feelings. David Mann (1997) suggests the astonishingly high number of therapists who do abuse might be because not only sexual contact but also thinking about sexual or erotic feelings in relation to clients is taboo. When something is forbidden in practice it also becomes repressed in thought, and when something is repressed the energy around it increases. Look what happened to poor Oedipus, who did everything possible to avoid transgressing the incest taboo and ended up doing just that, by marrying his own mother.

There is a great relief that comes from allowing discussion of the forbidden, or the unacceptable. This is the rationale behind support groups of all kinds. The feelings don't seem so terrible, the shame is lessened and ideas for coping are shared. But how many practitioners, of any persuasion, talk about getting turned on by a particular client, having lustful fantasies, or finding aspects of their work deeply erotic?

Sex and biology

Maybe it helps, at this point, to untangle the strands in the difficult and unavoidable subject of sex. There's the biological aspect, rooted in our brains, neural pathways and hormones, with one set of each for men and another for women and all kinds of permutations in between. Were it not for our social conditioning, taboos and prohibitions, or learning that delayed gratification can be preferable to here-and-now immediacy, biological arousal would lead automatically to sexual behaviour, including genital sex. If sexuality is understood as a biological fact, then arousal is just a physical response to certain stimuli and something that happens to all of us, man or woman, practitioner or client. We get turned on because we're human beings – it's proof that we're alive. In the same way that the sight and smell of a plate of delicious food makes our mouth water, contact with certain other people, depending on our preferences, can set off the neural circuits and trigger a rush of hormones that spell sex. Men who express concern that their penis might develop a mind of its own, so to speak, during a massage are only too aware of this connection. But because we are socialised human beings, we do not act on our biological arousal unless the circumstances are right.

Sex and sensuality

All sexual encounters include elements of sensuality, even those that seem exclusively genital, if sensuality is understood in its widest sense, as pertaining to the senses. The arousal phase of a sexual encounter, in particular, engages the tactile and kinaesthetic sense, as well as sight, smell, taste and hearing. Sensuality is not only a strand of sexuality certainly, but also an aspect of all pleasurable bodily experience. Remember how the sun feels on your face after a long winter, the smell of earth after rain, of coffee brewing, the softness of velvet, and the freshness of ironed cotton, chocolate melting in your mouth or the scrunch of a biscuit. Remember how it feels getting into a warm bath at the end of the day or touching the face of a tiny baby. These are sensual but not sexual experiences. I enjoy the sensuality in giving massage, the skin-on-skin contact, the feel of flesh moving under my hands, muscles releasing as I knead them. I get pleasure in my ability to coax, tease or soothe a body into a state of relaxation. I wouldn't do massage if I didn't get pleasure from it. But it isn't sexual. I wonder if my pleasure in the sensuality of it is self gratification? I don't think so, because I don't need my clients' bodies to satisfy my need for physical contact or pleasurable touch, having plenty of other circumstances in my personal life for that. I hope that my sensual pleasure in a client's body communicates to her a basic message that this is a good body and I appreciate it.

Sex as an expression of the life force

And then there are the forces of desire and longing, that arise internally but seek an external object for their satisfaction. In common with other mammals, we desire and look for things that will satisfy our biological needs: water if we are thirsty, shade if it's too hot, or a safe place to sleep when we are tired. But we have other desires, which aren't anything to do with sex. My nephew longs to play in a rock band, a friend has a dream of a pilgrimage to Peru and another is passionate about raising funds for Tibetan children in exile. These individual longings, based on a complex interaction of biological, emotional and spiritual forces, are manifestations of the life force. Freud placed sexuality at the centre of the life force and ever since we've had difficulty seeing it as anything else. Jung disagreed with Freud (Smith 1999, p.53), believing that creativity, as the expression of the soul on earth, had to be included as part of the life force. Eros, the Greek god who long preceded either of them, and whose name we recognise in the word erotic, was god not only of love and sex, but a personification of life energy. Eros, then, is a force that is part creative and part sexual. Sex is, after all, a desire to create new life, as Kahlil Gibran says, in *The Prophet*:

> Your children are not your children.
> They are the sons and daughters of Life's longing for itself. (1971, p.20)

From birth, the life force is subject to forces that shape, channel or suppress it. The aim of many complementary therapies is to remove these blocks that prevent full expression of the life force in an individual. The massage practitioner works with holding in the muscular armouring, the acupuncturist and the shiatsu practitioner balance energy in the meridians, osteopaths work with lesions in the tissues, craniosacral therapists with fulcrums in the fluid systems, healers with energy blockages in the chakra, homeopaths with the miasmas and so on. We work to restore health and vitality by allowing expression of the life force, whether it's called qi, prana or the breath of life. If sexual energy arises during a treatment, isn't this just an aspect of the life force? I think this quote from Jack Lee Rosenberg, author of *Body Self and Soul*, helps here:

> Many people believe that if they experience sexual energy they have to do something about it – perform, act it out, discharge it. Sexual energy is a function of being alive, all they have to do is experience it – contain and let it spread over the whole body. (1985, p.233)

The sexual vignettes discussed

In the examples at the beginning of this section, all four people reported a degree of sexual arousal with clients. In 'The Vampire Casanova', an imaginary story to illustrate how powerful sexual feelings can be not only allowed but also understood in a psychotherapeutic relationship, Susie Orbach (1999) describes the impact of the 'Casanova' in question, her patient, on her body when she was with him and on her fantasy life when she was not. She doesn't suppress her powerful physical sensations and dreams, nor does she think they are wrong, or inappropriate, but lets herself experience them, wondering what they can tell her about this particular man. It's part of her job, as a psychoanalyst, to let herself be affected by her patient. It's not the job of the complementary therapist. It happens, at times, that we experience feelings that we can't understand and then we look at what might be going on in the transference, but it's not our job to explore it with the client. But this story does tell us two important things: first, that sexual feelings in the therapeutic relationship aren't, per se, wrong; and, second, that they belong to the practitioner, and should not be discussed with the client. Susie Orbach makes this very clear. She never tells her 'Casanova' about her sexual feelings towards him. It is her business, as therapist, to contain and make sense of her feelings, and to act appropriately.

Gary, the massage therapist mentioned at the beginning of this chapter, was trying very hard to act appropriately as well. He didn't respond to sexual invitations from his first client or indicate that they were having any impact on him. He kept his arousal to himself. (Maybe he should have talked with the client about the inappropriateness of his behaviour, but that's another story.) But then he used the next client to discharge his sexual energy, without being explicitly sexual. No code of conduct was broken there, we could say. And yet he was using the client for his own means, and the therapeutic relationship should not be a place for self gratification. Of course none of us are completely free of our own needs when we meet a client. Apart from our need for financial compensation, we also have complex needs relating to self esteem, power, wanting to be of use, to care for others, to heal or to fix. These are powerful forces and I'm not sure if any therapeutic relationship can be completely free of the practitioner's desire for something, and need to have that desire gratified. But our patients or clients are not there to gratify our sexual desires or our need for intimacy. And that is why the healer who talked about increasing her own sexual pleasure during sessions is behaving inappropriately by using her male clients for her own purpose.

And what about James? Of course, it depends on whether James is the client or the practitioner. He finds himself aroused by his companion and, assuming he's a young male with healthy hormonal responses, there's nothing wrong with his biological reaction. If he's the client he's also at liberty to express what's happening in his body. If he's been asked about other aspects of his bodily functioning, why shouldn't he talk about this one too? But if he's the practitioner, then he has absolutely no business bringing his own feelings into the session. He can't prevent himself having the feelings but they are his own personal experience, and he has a professional responsibility to keep them to himself.

Sex in the therapeutic relationship: how to work safely

Sexual energy and life force energy are powerful forces and when aroused can engender fear; fear of change, of being overwhelmed by the feelings, fear of breaking taboos, losing touch with our rational adult selves and forgetting about codes of conduct and our responsibilities. How can we acknowledge sexual energy, our own or our clients', and stay within therapeutic boundaries, both professional and personal?

1. Remember, sex is an energy, it is not wrong and it does not have to be acted upon, just experienced. It is also the responsibility of the person experiencing it.

2. If the sexual feelings clearly belong to the client, see if it is possible to ascertain his or her intention. Be alert to things the client says which may indicate that his intention is to use the treatment as a sexual experience, as sometimes happens, particularly with massage. Terminate the session, and/or be explicit about boundaries. State that you do not offer sexual contact.

3. A client may have sexual feelings as a response to treatment, which are just part of what's happening – a biological response or an energetic release. If this happens (and I'm not saying that it's easy to differentiate between intentional sexual responses and unintentional ones) and you feel able to accept this, don't shame or blame the client, and if necessary state your boundaries, to remind both of you of the safety of the relationship. I sometimes say, 'It's all right to have sexual feelings and you know that nothing sexual will happen here between us.'

4. If you aren't comfortable with clients' sexual feelings then refer them on. It isn't good practice to work outside your comfort zone. Talk to colleagues, or your supervisor.

5. Sometimes it just isn't clear where the feelings belong. If there is sexual energy around, you may be picking it up, a form of somatic resonance or physical empathy. Try these tools to sort out what's going on: refocus your own intention on the work you are doing, on your purpose with the client. If you work with energy, acknowledge the feelings and let them go into the earth. If you normally talk with your client during the treatment, you could try asking what's going on for them, what are they feeling? Sometime naming something helps disperse it.

6. If you've tried the above and the feelings are is still there, or you find yourself thinking sexually about a client outside of sessions, again, you're not doing anything wrong. Yet. Risk factors for therapists who do abuse include having sexual thoughts and feelings about clients, in conjunction with social isolation or going through a period of distress or crisis. If either of those applies, or you find yourself taking more care of your appearance with a certain client, going over time, being lenient about money, talking about yourself more than usual, flirting and not talking about this client in supervision, then you are at risk of inappropriate sexual behaviour.

7. What to do? If possible, stop working with the client (and read the following section on sex with former clients). Get help; talk to a senior colleague or find a supervisor. Remind yourself of your professional responsibilities by reading your professional code of conduct. Try an affirmation such as 'There's nothing wrong with sexual feelings but I do not have sexual contact with clients.' And, finally, find more ways to get your needs for contact and intimacy met in your personal life.

Sex and former clients

I've discussed the taboo against sex between practitioner and client while they are engaged in a therapeutic relationship, but the issue about sex with former clients is one that requires more thought. Codes of ethics don't always tell us what to do about sexual contact after a professional relationship ends. I was curious what my colleagues might have to say about this, so I emailed 30 colleagues, psychotherapists, CAM practitioners and some, like myself, working in both fields; 25 replied. The questions were:

1. Is it OK to have sex with former clients?

2. If so, under what circumstances?

I anticipated that the psychotherapists would say no and CAM practitioners yes and to some extent the results confirmed that guess, but there was also a large proportion who weren't able to say clearly one way or another, and admitted that they had to think about it.

The five psychotherapists and one CAM practitioner who believed that sex with former clients was never acceptable gave much clearer reasons for their answer than those who thought it might be permissible, sometimes or in certain circumstances. One psychotherapist sums these reasons up when she says:

I don't think that it is OK to have sex with a former client for these reasons:

1. The therapist has to be very respectful of the power imbalance implicit in the therapeutic relationship (of any kind, whether medical or psychological therapy). This client entered the relationship in the trust they would not be used for the practitioner's own emotional or physical needs. The contract that they enter into is not socially interpersonal, but bound by professional ethics.

2. It is hard to imagine how this relationship could be sufficiently revised over time for that power imbalance to ever be completely resolved. Even if the treatment has long since ended the relational dynamic will be embedded in non-equal structures.

3. Non-equal structures (doctor–patient, teacher–student, etc.) are part of a parent–child paradigm.

4. Finally, the patient may need to resume treatment in the future. What then?

And Anthony, a body psychotherapist and massage practitioner, echoes this:

I believe it is never right for a complementary therapist to have sex with a former client. I am writing this from the standpoint of a therapist for whom the relationship is central and for whom there is always an emotional component in the work. The issue is one of the vulnerability of the client in the client–therapist relationship and this leads to distorted perceptions, which may never go away. However much work is done to ensure a balance of power, this is never fully achieved. It is only because there is no possibility of there *ever* being a sexual relationship with the therapist that the client can safely explore his/her sexual feelings for the therapist knowing the boundary will always be preserved.

At the other end of the spectrum, five CAM practitioners (and no psychotherapists) saw no problem as long as the professional relationship had ended. 'Work and personal life should always be kept separate, and whatever happens after that is about mutual choice.'

But most were of the opinion that the dynamics of the professional relationship could, perhaps, transfer into a sexual one if certain conditions were met. Five psychotherapists and nine CAM practitioners thought that it would be acceptable under certain circumstances. Time was the factor mentioned most often, the idea being that allowing a time lapse between a professional and personal relationship would somehow do the trick, but that this would be hard to legislate and even harder to monitor. David le May, massage practitioner, points this out:

...should a practitioner meet a former client socially ten years after the professional relationship had ended, and they were to become mutually attracted, a proscription on a personal relationship between them surely would be absurd. On the other hand, should they meet socially on the day after the professional relationship had ended, and feel mutually attracted, the start of a personal relationship at that time would surely be inappropriate as it would seem to arise directly out of the professional one.

Andy Fagg, director of the Bristol College of Massage and Bodywork, offered clear guidelines:

> My guidelines on developing a personal relationship with a former client are that the therapeutic relationship should finish first. Then a period of no contact for a good six months and only then explore whether a personal relationship is both desired and desirable.

Five respondents mentioned the power imbalance, transference and projection and the need for these to be worked through first, but without proposing how to do this, and three mentioned that it might depend on the nature of the professional relationship.

> The more intimate the therapy e.g. body work, massage etc. and the longer the therapy the more dubious I would be.
> I would be open to the argument that a therapist whose work is largely mechanical might at some period after the ending of their therapeutic contract be open harmlessly to exploring relationships of another kind.

And a number suggested the importance of the practitioner getting professional support before entering into a sexual relationship.

> I recommended seeking professional help before making a decision.
> It is absolutely necessary for the therapist to consult a senior practitioner and his/her professional body.

Conclusions

In my survey some practitioners (six) said sex with former clients was never acceptable, a few (five) thought that as long as the professional relationship had ended, there was no problem and the majority (14) that it might be permissible if certain conditions were met. These included a 'cooling off' period and talking about the attraction in supervision or with colleagues. The nature of the therapeutic relationship was also a factor mentioned, with shorter, more mechanistic, or non-touch therapies considered less of a problem for the development of an emotional transference.

However, if psychotherapists, who are trained to work with these matters, are sometimes unclear about the difference between transference feelings and real feelings, surely it is much more difficult for complementary therapists, who are not trained in this area, to judge. Psychotherapists, on the other hand, are generally of the opinion that the power dynamic set up during a professional relationship endures so maybe we should always be very cautious when we consider sexual relationships with former clients and if in doubt, as one person said, 'Do the loving thing and abstain.'

Psychotherapy and the Therapeutic Relationship

Over time, psychotherapy and, in particular, psychoanalysis, which is one branch of psychotherapy, or maybe more accurately the trunk from which all other branches grew, has developed a repertoire of concepts and ways of thinking about our inner worlds, how they might function, how our inner world is affected by events in the outer world, particularly how this affects our relationships with others. Some of the words that psychoanalysts use are now part of our everyday language. It's hard to imagine, for example, that only 200 years ago, the idea that we had something called an unconscious didn't exist. Possibly more has been written about Freud, and what he really meant, than about any of the great twentieth-century thinkers, and there is no doubt that his work changed our thinking.

Let's suppose you decide to go and see a psychoanalyst. He or she will use his or her understanding of psychoanalytic concepts as tools to treat your problem, in the same way that many complementary therapists use their hands as tools to treat a problem. Your analyst will also focus on the relationship between the two of you in the consulting room as a means of attending to difficulties in your inner world. This is where the term 'the therapeutic relationship' originated, in this form of psychotherapy that actually uses the relationship between therapist and patient as the medium in which healing occurs. All schools of psychotherapy today have either grown directly out of Freud's legacy, or owe him some debt.

This chapter will attempt to explain some psychotherapy terms as simply as possible, together with a little about the historical context in which they emerged. Remember, they are only ideas, not necessarily right or wrong, but ideas that can offer us a framework for looking at our inner worlds and the relationships we have with other people, including those we work with, just as the anatomical model of the body, homeopathic pictures, the chakra system, and the seven elements of traditional Chinese medicine (TCM) are also frameworks that explain particular phenomena.

A brief history: how psychoanalysis began

Psychotherapy began in the late 1880s. Sigmund Freud qualified as a doctor in Vienna and because he was Jewish found himself allocated the patients no one wanted to work with, people with psychiatric problems. He became fascinated in the relationship between the mind and the body and began his investigations into mental suffering as a neurologist, convinced that the problems lay in the brain and nerves, but, since the equipment available at the time was quite inadequate to the task of such study, he gave up in this area and devoted himself to developing a framework of the mind that was purely conceptual and had no relation to the physical reality of the body. In fact such was the force with which the new science of psychotherapy rejected physical reality that Wilhelm Reich, who continued to maintain the centrality of the body in therapy, and whose ideas underpin the work of most body therapists today, was thrown out of the Vienna analytical society which developed around Freud and his ideas.

Having abandoned the anatomical path, Freud began to use his own mind (or psyche) as a tool for understanding what was happening in the minds of his patients. His hypothesis was that somatic symptoms might have their origin in the psyche, and that if the underlying problem was brought to light and understood, the physical manifestation of it would disappear. 'The talking cure', as it came to be called, depended on the analyst, sitting behind the patient who lay on a couch, allowing his mind to empty while the patient talked. The analyst's job wasn't to respond to the patient but to 'interpret' what he was talking about according to the Freudian model. By now we are all so sophisticated that we know that references to pencils, corn cobs and candles mean that someone is talking about a penis; and shoes, cups and bowls scattered about in conversation are references to vaginas. But seriously, although we can now understand why Freud put sexuality at the core of his theories, growing up in a sexually repressive middle-class era, he was the first person to suggest that the superficial content of what someone says might not be the whole story, and that if we listen carefully, there may be other meanings in the communication.

Although these days many of his Freud's original ideas have been revised, replaced or discredited by later analysts, there are several key concepts which are not only employed by all kinds of psychotherapists but have also filtered into everyday usage. Let's have a look at them.

Key concepts

The unconscious

In Freud's map of the mind, there were three zones: one conscious, one preconscious and the other unconscious. The conscious mind contains all that the person is aware of in the here and now, the thoughts in his head, the feelings from his body and impressions from the outside world. The preconscious mind contains all that isn't immediately conscious but could become so quite easily. This includes memory. If you were asked what you did last night or to recite the two times table you'd manage, it is hoped, to find the information somewhere. Freud called this somewhere the preconscious. The unconscious is that part of the psyche that contains everything that has been buried out of conscious reach and can't be remembered under ordinary circumstances. Freud believed that some memories were thrust into the unconscious because they were unbearable. He developed a technique called free association, which meant that the patient said whatever came into his mind in response to words spoken by the analyst, as a means of revealing the troublesome contents of the unconscious, bringing them into the light for analysis and understanding. In everyday usage, a Freudian slip occurs when someone says something without meaning to, which might reveal an unconscious thought. If a guest says to his hostess 'Thanks for forcing me to come' as he leaves a party he didn't really want to go to, he's inadvertently communicating his true feelings about the party. But not all of the silly verbal mistakes we make are Freudian slips; they really are only mistakes and nothing else.

An unconscious communication refers to something that is said which might seem out of context or irrelevant but might also be conveying a message to the listener. Here's an example. When Marie arrived for her session I could hear that she'd passed a couple of people on the stairs. She started by telling me about her bus journey, how the bus had been so full she'd had to stand all the way, how much she hated being squashed. I knew she came from a family of 12 children. When I suggested that she might be worried that I might not have room for her she smiled and relaxed. This showed me that I'd been correct in guessing that she was talking about what had just happened to her, but also, without knowing it, about her childhood experience of being one among many.

The superego

Living in the sexually repressive atmosphere of nineteenth-century Vienna, Freud placed sexual anxiety at the core of his theories. He invented the concepts of the id, ego and superego to explain how people manage the conflict between their inherent animal natures, as he saw it, and their social selves. According to him, the id is the part of the psyche where powerful instinctual forces reside. The superego develops in order to keep a check on these antisocial forces. The ego is the day-to-day self, the one we identify with and call our self; it's the face we present to the world. The superego is the one that we can all relate to. The concept has filtered down in different guises through the humanistic psychotherapies, called by names like the inner judge, the internal critic or the censor. Often containing things that we were told as part of growing up by parents and teachers in their attempts to train and socialise us, the role of this part of our inner world is to make sure we don't get into trouble, draw attention to ourselves, get too big for our boots and so on. When the inner judge is too ferocious or overzealous, we find ourselves lacking in confidence, with low self worth and rather rigid in our behaviour. The inner judge does not care for spontaneity.

Most of us have a pretty strong inner judge or critic, a voice inside which whispers a litany of our faults to prevent us from getting too big headed. If we really do make a mistake, the volume is turned up to full blast. 'You're *so* stupid! Only you could mess up big time like that! Why didn't you think properly?' Does this sound familiar? A close friend of the inner critic is the inner censor, the part of our self which is so convinced that the whole world is going to attack us for what we think or say that it prevents us from opening our mouths or putting pen to paper. Another acquaintance is the inner saboteur, whose litany goes something like this: 'It's no good. This won't work. Why do I even bother? Might as well give up now.'

Once upon a time these voices were outside our heads. The phrases we use to police our thoughts and behaviours were probably said to us at one time by a parent, older sibling or a teacher. Someone whose goodwill we relied on, someone we trusted, a big person who, if she said we were stupid, we had no reason to doubt. As children we internalised these phrases to pre-empt the big people saying them to us. If we could learn to monitor what we did, we wouldn't get into trouble. A sensible approach, but one that is effective for a five year old may not be much help to a 35 year old.

These kinds of thoughts affect us. When we think negative, we feel negative. Scientists have discovered a physical reality behind this statement. Positive thoughts actually stimulate the release of neurochemicals in the brain that are associated with good feelings, and self-critical thoughts stem the flow of these chemicals. The position of our skeletal muscles, and our bones, also determines how we feel. Try this: move the little muscle around your mouth into a smile and notice sensations that arise in your chest, heart area and upper body. How does smiling make you feel? Here's another experiment. Wherever you are sitting as you read, let your spine collapse, your shoulders sag forwards and your head drop. What happens? Now pull your spine erect, look forwards and roll your shoulders back and down. Feel different? Negative self-thinking is often reflected in a collapsed posture.

Inner critic exercise

Here's an experiment to try with a friend. You each need writing materials. Divide your paper into two columns. In one column write a list of all your own negative, self-hating, self-blaming thoughts. Swap papers. On your friend's paper look at the statements he or she has written and next to each one in the other column write the opposite, or a positive phrase that gives the opposite message. For example, if one of the critical thoughts is 'I'm so ugly' try writing 'You're a very attractive person.' 'I'm lazy' could be transformed to 'You appreciate the need to get good rest.' When you've both finished take it in turns to first read out loud to the other several times his or her critical thoughts. As the listener, notice how you feel inside listening to all that stuff. Pay attention to your body. Don't answer back, just listen. When you have both had a turn hearing your own critical thoughts read out loud, take it in turns to read the other, positive list. Again, notice what happens inside listening to all the good things. How does it feel to hear affirmative statements about you? Which list is easier to listen to?

Transference

Transference means, literally, 'to carry across'. Freud's early patients for his new psychoanalytic technique were often young women with troubled histories. He realised that they often developed strong feelings for him, both negative and positive, and came to understand these feelings as being transferred from another important person in his patients' life onto himself. In the psychoanalytic branch of psychotherapy, the patient transfers onto the analyst intense loving or hateful thoughts and feelings from earlier important relationships, notably parental ones. Psychoanalysts believe that the suffering resulting from dysfunctional early relationships can be alleviated by a re-enactment between analyst and patient leading to a more satisfactory resolution. This term is used somewhat loosely by psychotherapists these days, and has come to mean any feelings that the client might have about the therapist, both those transferred from someone else as well as those that do belong with the analyst himself or herself.

In everyday life transference operates in many of our interactions. Here's an example. My friend Arthur works in a health practice where most of the other practitioners are women, and older than him. He finds staff meetings very difficult because he often experiences their comments as criticism. He was the youngest child, and his three older sisters teased and criticised him for not keeping up with their games. He 'transfers' onto older women the expectations and fear that he'll still be found wanting.

HELEN'S STORY: AN EXAMPLE OF TRANSFERENCE

Helen was one of my psychotherapy clients who developed a powerful positive transference. Her mother had died when she was about four and she often told me how she remembered watching the car that took her mother away. She never came back. For Helen, it was as if I was the wonderful loving mother that she had lost. She transferred feelings about her mother onto me, her therapist, both her love and pleasure but also her intense anxiety that I, too, would die and leave her. At our first meeting she began to cry, and said: 'I'm imagining the time when we will say goodbye and I feel so sad.' This before we had even got to know each other! The holidays were always very difficult times, which Helen coped with by leaving me. About three weeks before the break she would announce that she was better and didn't need to come anymore, and I would say that I'd keep her session time after the holiday, just in case she changed her mind. Which she always did. I hadn't done anything to warrant these feelings apart from being someone prepared to spend time listening to her and attending to her feelings, and someone who left her to have holidays. I think Helen eventually learned to trust that I would return, something she never managed with her real mother.

Countertransference

The feelings that a therapist has towards the client are called counter-transference feelings. Initially Freud believed that any feelings he had towards his patients were wrong and a failure of his professional neutrality, but over time other analysts came to realise that countertransference was an important part of the work, because these feelings provide information about what is occurring in the relationship. Sometimes, as the example below shows, a countertransference reaction is entirely to do with the client. When this happens the therapist may be surprised or puzzled by the responses she has to her client, because they may not make any sense. But countertransference can also include the analyst's own feelings that are triggered by the patient. When Joan developed a cataract and was waiting for a lens transplant operation, one of her clients described taking her father to hospital for the same operation, which had failed, badly, leaving him partially sighted. Joan was well aware that the agitation she felt listening to her client's anger was partly motivated by concerns for her own future well being as well as being a countertransference reaction to her client.

GEORGE AND THE DISGUSTING CLIENT: AN EXAMPLE OF COUNTERTRANSFERENCE

George, an osteopath, was puzzled by a strong aversion he experienced to touching one of his patients, a pleasant, intelligent, expensively dressed woman in her forties. She was clean, had no physical deformity or any other sign that might evoke such a response. Being an experienced professional, he was able to put his reactions on one side while he treated her. During the third session she told him about an accident she'd had as a child. The resulting wound had turned septic, oozing, as she put it 'disgusting green smelly pus' which had caused her mother to retch each time she changed the dressing. George made some comment like 'That must have been horrible for you.' The incident wasn't discussed again, but George's aversion vanished and he understood it as a non-verbal and unconscious communication from his patient about her concern that he too would find her body disgusting and smelly.

SOMATIC COUNTER TRANSFERENCE

Freud and the early psychoanalysts understood emotions to be mental constructs, to do with thinking processes (the psyche) rather than the body (soma). The relationship between psychoanalysis and the body has always been a tenuous one, partly because of the mistakes which caused several analysts to confuse intense transference–countertransference feelings with the real thing, resulting in seductions and sexual relationships, and partly because of the mind–body split in Western thinking and medical practice. Mind and its contents were understood to be separate stuff to the body. Today it is recognised that emotions originate in the body, associated with certain visceral responses, tightening of muscles (particularly in the face, neck and throat) and release of certain neurochemicals into the blood. Arriving at the brain, these signals activate particular neural pathways and brain sites, which are the templates, as it were, for feelings, and finally other brain sites recognise the feelings. An emotion that is not strong enough to enter consciousness is called a mood, a pervasive background feeling (Damasio 2000). So we could say that all countertransference, all the feelings that arise in the practitioner in relation to the client, are somatic countertransference.

FALLING ASLEEP WITH A CLIENT: SOMATIC COUNTERTRANSFERENCE

I experienced a particularly striking period of somatic countertransference while I was seeing Marion for psychotherapy for depression and feeling stuck in her life. During the second year that we were working together I found myself becoming incredibly sleepy in the sessions, so much so that it was hard to keep my eyes open and to stop myself yawning. I also had twitching sensations in my legs, which wanted to jerk and kick. This happened around four o'clock, which I know can be a metabolic low point for me, but it didn't occur with other clients that I saw at that time on other days. Not knowing what to make of it or how to talk to Marion about it, I waited. Over the weeks she slowly revealed what she saw as terrible secrets, things she thought about that she knew meant she was a very bad person. Her conviction that I wouldn't approve and would judge her, or, worse, say that I couldn't work with her anymore, was so strong that she communicated this to me by sending me to sleep, as it were, so that I couldn't think about her. Every time she managed to confess one of her secrets I would become alert and awake and my sleepy feelings just vanished. Over time I could begin to talk to her about the effect she was having on me until it got to the point that, when I started to feel sleepy, I could ask her if there was something she was having trouble talking about.

✍ Somatic countertransference exercise

Somatic countertransference refers to all the feelings that a practitioner has about a client. This exercise helps you explore and possibly identify those feelings. You'll need a quiet uninterrupted space and writing materials. Sit quietly and let your mind settle. Focus on your breathing for a few moments. Do whatever you usually do to become grounded, centred and still.

Begin to think about the person. Bring him to mind; maybe imagining him standing in front of you, or as you last saw him in your treatment room. If visualising is hard for you, go through the last session in your mind, remembering your conversations and the treatment you gave. As you do this, allow part of your attention to monitor what's happening in your body. Notice sensations in your guts, changes to your breathing, to your heart rate and to tension in your muscles. As you watch the sensations see if there are words or phrases that come to mind to describe your feelings. Write them down here, without thinking too hard about them. Just write.

Now look at what you've written and consider your somatic countertransference in the light of these questions, which are intended to offer guidelines, not definitive answers.

1. Does any of it make sense to you?
2. Do any of your feelings correspond to what you may know about your client's past history?
3. Do any of your feelings correspond to what you may know about your client's body/symptoms?
4. Do these feelings remind you of anything? Are they familiar from another situation?
5. If your body could speak, what might it be trying to communicate through these feelings?

Here are the experiences of two people who did this exercise, which illustrate some of the psychotherapeutic ideas described earlier.

SALLY AND HER DIFFICULT CLIENT

Sally visualised a woman, a psychotherapy client, that she found very difficult because of the push and pull dynamic between them. Sometimes her client thought she was truly wonderful, and at other times, when Sally made a 'mistake', the adoration turned to hate. When Sally brought her attention back to herself in this exercise, she was struck by a tight heavy feeling in her neck and across her shoulders. As she focused on it the thought came to her: 'I'm being crucified'. She realised that, at times, that was exactly what she felt like. Looking back at her client, she described a sense of spaciousness around her heart and then a sudden brief image of Sally kicking her client. Again, she recognised she did feel like this at times. But, knowing how much the other woman had been bullied as a child, she could also see it as a message from the client about her concern that Sally would end up 'kicking her when she was down' just like everyone else.

The somatic sensations were about both the therapist's own feelings of frustration, and also contained elements communicated from the client.

JO AND HER DIFFICULT CLIENT

Doing the exercise, Jo had strong physical sensations and thoughts which she described as follows: 'There's lots of anger, I'm strangled, my jaw's clenched, who's most angry here? I can't swallow, I feel choked, he's overmothering me, wants me to do it his way. He's just like my mother, oh he's very similar, even though he's not the same sex'. At this point Jo, a body psychotherapist, recognised her transference onto her client, who, even though he was male, reminded her strongly of her mother, and evoked in her the same responses she felt towards her mother. She found the exercise very helpful because, in her words, 'I merge easily with other people, and doing this helped me to pull back from him, and look at my own reactions. When I did this, I got my power back, and it was easy to see what I needed to say to him'.

Splitting

Melanie Klein was an analyst who trained with Freud and then developed her own theories abut the development of the psyche in newborn babies, who are possessed of extremely intense feelings, which they have no capacity to make sense of, or the ability to manage or contain. Anyone who has witnessed a little baby screaming knows the strength of feeling behind the screams, as well as the strength of response that this can elicit in the hearer. Melanie Klein postulated (Smith 1999, Ch.10) that the way the baby manages her feelings is to separate them out into feelings that make the baby feel good (full tummy, falling asleep on mother's body) and those that make her feel bad and seem to threaten her survival (tummy pain, feeling too cold, missing mother's body). The psychotherapeutic term for this mechanism is splitting. This is where the term 'the bad breast' comes from. Many babies do seem to show a preference for one breast over the other when feeding, and Klein suggested that the baby sees one as all good, loving and nurturing and the other as bad, destructive and poisonous. The developmental task facing the baby is to recognise that good and bad exist alongside each other, that her mother, the other important adults and even the baby herself are capable of being both good and bad. Remember, this is a psychoanalytic construct, and whether or not small babies' minds do work in that way, the concept of splitting is a useful one, as we shall see.

Splitting is not confined to babies. In this story, a small incident manages to destroy a person's sense of well being. Julie had arranged a special dinner at a favourite restaurant, to celebrate her husband's return from a successful business trip. She had her hair done, dressed with care and really wanted the evening to go well. During the meal she accidentally spilt a little wine on her dress and suddenly her mood changed. The food was bland, the restaurant stuffy, she was sure her husband was bored, and the whole evening was ruined. Unable to hold the possibility of good and bad together in her inner world, Julie's spoilt dress meant that everything was spoilt. The evening was all good or all bad, with nothing in between.

Projection

Projection is a mixture of transference and splitting. Put very simply, we separate ourselves from characteristics, attitudes, values and traits that we can't tolerate or admit to in ourselves and transfer them to another person. In the cinema, images are projected onto a blank screen. In life, we human beings project images, usually an amalgamation from our personal, social and cultural histories, onto other people. Some of these projections might 'fit', in the sense that what we imagine to be true about a person we meet might really be so, but other projections might be just that, an idea from our own mind with no relation to the person. In the cinema, we're supposed to watch the image projected but in life the more we can own and take back our projections, the easier it is to see the screen, the real person behind them.

I remember learning a lesson about projection. In my feminist youth I was once paired up in a workshop with the man I disliked the most in the group. I had no reason to dislike him: I didn't know anything about him. But since he was white, middle aged, dressed in a good quality suit and had other accoutrements of success like a Rolex and a leather briefcase, he automatically attracted all my projections about men at that time. He had to be egotistical, selfish, insensitive (though what he'd be doing in a personal development workshop if he was all these things hadn't occurred to me) and very sexist. The exercise was to take it in turns to talk about some issue, I forget what, while the other listened. I hated him so much that I couldn't look at him while I was talking. I finished. Silence. I looked up and, to my surprise, saw compassion in his eyes. My projection was shattered in that moment. I was looking at a caring, compassionate man and not the monster I'd imagined him to be.

The shadow

Carl Gustav Jung was one of Freud's students who developed his own systems of thinking about the mind. One of his contributions (Jung 1993) was to suggest that the psyche contains a shadow, a part that we can't see, that isn't available to consciousness. Like the face of the moon, part of our mind is in the light and part is in the darkness. Based on the belief that we all have the potential to be anything, our shadow self tends to contain those aspects that we most dislike or fear about ourselves, these parts we want to disown. Note that the shadow doesn't always contain negative human qualities. Within the shadow of a mass murderer might be found love and compassion for suffering. As Caroline Myss, talking about the shadow side of the healer points out, it isn't negative, but unknown and very hard to own up to, if it does surface (Myss 2004). Healers tend to identify with their role with the spiritual path, with connotations of suffering martyrdom and self denial, she says, but the flip side may be an attraction to the drama of illness and the glory and applause that comes with an ability to make things better. She also says that healers often believe that their hypersensitivity makes them special and different from other people. The shadow side of such specialness is the belief that no other healers are as good, or able to help their clients as well.

Jung suggested three different aspects to the shadow: personal, collective and archetypal. The personal shadow is a collection of memories, images, forbidden desires and so on that have to be suppressed for personal reasons. The collective shadow contains all that is unacceptable in a group, be it a family, organisation, town, country or nation, and the archetypal shadow contains the energy that drives the other two kinds. The drive behind all shadow aspects is to destroy the good and ideal in the individual or group, so the more that the shadow can be accepted, the less power it has. As Adolf Guggenbuhl-Craig (1971) says, 'Only the possibility of destroying the world can enable us to love it.'

✍ **Exercise to explore your personal shadow**
Although it isn't possible to grasp your shadow self (did you ever try to step on your shadow when you were a child?) this simple exercise gives a taste of what might be lurking in yours. Make two columns on a page. In one, write a list of your most important qualities and characteristics, the things you really like about yourself, the things you are proud of. Some of these attributes you may have been born with and some you may have struggled hard to cultivate. Don't think too hard about it. Now, next to each word or phrase, write the opposite. If you described yourself as kind, thoughtful and responsible, the opposite would be unkind, unthinking, and irresponsible. The second list may contain parts of yourself that you've relegated to your shadow, your unwanted negative self that it is easier to disown.

Something we all tend to do is project our split-off characteristics onto others. It's much more comfortable to agree with statements like 'suicide bombers are mad' than it is to consider our own potential for random destruction. This kind of projection underlies all the –isms you can think of. Racism, sexism, ageism and the others all exist because groups of people identify other groups as different, which they are, but then project onto that difference qualities that make the other group inferior, not as good as or, in some way, bad. It's natural to feel comfortable with people like ourselves, people with a shared background and a similar outlook on life.

In the Danish film *In Your Hands* (Oleson 2004) a newly ordained priest, Anna, finds herself working in a prison. One of the inmates, Kate, has a reputation as a healer with the ability to help women withdraw from drugs almost miraculously. Anna is very sceptical about all things 'New Age'. Kate is in prison for allowing her baby daughter to die of thirst when she went out on a drug bender and didn't come home for four days. When Anna finds herself pregnant with a potentially deformed foetus, she and her boyfriend have to decide whether or not to terminate the pregnancy. The night before the termination Anna goes to the prison and bursts into Kate's cell, pleading for her help. Kate slowly reaches out to Anna's stomach, but after a few moments Anna starts screaming at her that she knows what she did, and who does she think she is to help anyone. The priest, the person identified with god, goodness and the possibility of forgiveness, which we see her preaching on several occasions, reveals her shadow side at this moment; the part of herself she cannot accept, the part that is totally lacking in compassion and forgiveness, as she is about to murder her own baby.

Discovering your projections

If our thoughts affect our own bodies so can they also impact on other peoples.' Rupert Sheldrake is a biologist who has spent many years researching, among other things, telepathy. In his book *The Sense of Being Stared At* (2003) he describes a very simple experiment that he has carried out all over the world with all kinds of people, in all kinds of situations. What he discovered was this: if you stare at the back of someone's head, the likelihood that he or she will turn round is much higher than chance. Sheldrake proposes that the activity of our minds extends outside our heads, as an energetic field, so it is as if our minds can reach out to touch the person we are thinking about. And this brings an almost tangible reality to the psychotherapeutic concept of projections. So it can be helpful to examine your projections about different groups of people, since these may be influencing, in a very subtle way, how you react if someone from one of these groups happens to walk into your treatment room.

Exercise to explore projections

To discover some of your projections, try this. You must be prepared not to censor your thoughts, to accept anything that comes into your mind, to allow yourself to write things that you wouldn't dream of telling anyone. You can burn the paper when you've finished! So, without stopping, finish the following sentences.

Fat people are…
Old people are…
Black people are …
Men are …
Working class people are…
Transsexuals are…
Muslims are…
Jews are…
Drug users are…
People in wheelchairs are…
People with cancer are…
Middle-class people are…
Asylum seekers are…
Gay men are…
Christians are…
White people are…
Women are…
The young are…
People who are unemployed are…
Alcoholics are…
Lesbians are …

If, when you've done this exercise and reflected on the outcome, you recognise that there are some projections that might make it difficult for you to work with certain groups, you could think about talking to your supervisor, or treat it as a CPD project, and look for books or workshops that could further your learning.

✎ **Projections and individual clients**
One exercise to explore difficulties in relation to a particular client is to look at the projections you may be holding about him or her. Take some paper and without censoring, thinking too hard or stopping, write down all your thoughts about this person. Kind ones, cruel ones, even the totally politically incorrect thoughts that you would never admit to anyone else. Carry on until you dry up. Ask yourself if there's any more to come. You might, at this point, be blocking the most difficult projection of all, the one you really don't want to admit to yourself.

When you've finished, put the writing things down, stand up and do something else for a moment. Look out of the window, make a cup of tea, and look at your e-mails. This puts some distance between you and your thoughts about this person. Come back to your writing and put yourself in the other person's shoes. See if you can imagine that you are that person. Then read aloud all the things on the paper, as if they are being said to you, as the other person. What does it feel like to hear these things? Notice your reactions, your physical response, your thoughts, and any emotions that surface.

Projections about complementary therapists

Of course, projections work both ways; trouble with a client might be caused by a projection from the practitioner who, in turn, might be the subject of a projection from the client. Physical attributes, from height, body size and colour of skin to gesture and facial expression can trigger memory and associated feelings and beliefs related to significant other people in the client or practitioner's past or present life. The flow of information within the therapeutic relationship is more one way than the other, from client to practitioner. The client has less opportunity to make reality checks about his projections, to ask questions about the personal life or inner world of his practitioner, and find out who he really is, whereas the practitioner can and, depending on the sort of therapy, does do that.

All of us have been in the position of client at one time or another and may remember projections we've carried about professionals we've visited. I once caught myself, while travelling home after a wonderful Thai yoga massage, day dreaming about having a romantic dinner with the practitioner. My friend Julia says that she realised some way into her psychotherapy that a part of her had assumed that her therapist would make her better and then they'd get married. Isabel was devastated when she discovered that her lovely, bubbly cheerful homeopath who she saw in her beautiful home was a recovering alcoholic. Her image of the perfect person was broken by the news.

Projections can occur between professionals as well. Dan is a massage practitioner who works in a practice with other complementary therapists. At the last weekly team meeting a new osteopath had been introduced to the team. Dan had felt threatened by this man, and wanted to hide away. He used the somatic countertransference exercise. Visualising him, he saw a large, strong, self-confident man. When he came back to himself in the exercise, to his surprise, he also felt large, strong and self contained and recognised that he didn't need to be affected by this man. For some reason, Dan had projected these feelings onto the new osteopath, and experienced himself as diminished by comparison. In the exercise, he withdrew his projection, and allowed himself to feel strong and self-contained again.

Probably the most prevalent and collective projection that practitioners face at the moment derives from a splitting between traditional allopathic medicine and complementary therapy. The term 'alternative medicine', though not so widely used, fosters this splitting, suggesting as it does an either–or approach to healing. There are those in the complementary world, both practitioners and clients, who for various reasons including negative personal experience of traditional medicine, or because they hold radically different beliefs about the nature of healing, split the healing world into good complementary therapies and bad medical doctors, consultants and hospitals.

Anna was one such person who came to see me for craniosacral therapy for a temporo-mandibular joint problem. She was angry, and understandably so, with the dentist whose poor technique had dislocated her jaw, and with her doctor and the neurologist she'd been referred to, who not only found no cause for her headaches, insomnia and pain when eating but had seemed to her unsympathetic. 'They thought I was a trouble maker,' she said. 'I've given up on that lot. I know the answer lies in alternatives and so I've come to you. My friend says you can fix anything.' All of which made me very uncomfortable. I couldn't agree with her condemnation of the whole medical profession, but had to find a way to sympathise with her experience. I also had to be very clear about the possible outcomes using craniosacral therapy with her, and that I couldn't promise to fix her.

The scapegoat

There's a particular form of projection that occurs in groups. The scapegoat was a goat that was driven off into the wilderness as part of the ceremonies of

Yom Kippur, the Day of Atonement, in Judaism in ancient times. The goat carried away with it the sins of the community. Today scapegoating happens when an individual, or group, or nation, is blamed for a misfortune. On an unconscious level the group doing the scapegoating are projecting their feelings about the event onto the chosen scapegoat, so that they can feel better.

I remember one large and very diverse group of students that I took through a professional massage training. As often happens, there were more women than men. Of the five men in the group, one was blind, one was an eastern European refugee with broken English and one, let's call him Bill, was black British and older than the others. As the course went on, I noticed that individual women were coming to me to complain about Bill. He was looking at women while they were changing; he put his hand on someone's breast while massaging her neck; he kept his eyes open and watched when he was receiving massage. Several women felt strongly enough to have him excluded. I took these complaints seriously, although I had no sense myself that there was anything suspicious about Bill's behaviour. Observation of him in class confirmed this. Although he was a bit clumsy at times, he didn't show inappropriate interest in, or behaviour towards, the women in the group. I was puzzled. It wasn't until much later, after the group had graduated, that it dawned on me what had been happening. I suspect that the men that the women in the group really felt uncomfortable with, and didn't want to practise massage with, were the blind student and the refugee. But to express negative thoughts about these two so obviously disadvantaged students would have been impossible, so they were projected instead on to poor old Bill, who had been made a scapegoat for the difficult feelings that the women in the group couldn't express directly.

Archetypes

Jung's map of the mind contains two kinds of unconscious: the personal and the collective. The personal unconscious is that part of an individual's own consciousness which contains memories, fantasies, wishes and beliefs – and the shadow – which are not currently in their conscious awareness. Some of this material can be retrieved quickly, as in 'tell me what you did yesterday' or 'describe your childhood home', and some is much less accessible, and encountered in dreams, images and through creative writing or painting. The other kind, the collective unconscious, is the shared unconscious of a group; from the family to the nation, from a training organisation to a race, any kind of group could be said to have an unconscious aspect shared by all members of that group, which they may not be able to tap into, but which certainly influences the group. Within the collective unconsciousness are the archetypes, the blueprints for certain aspects of human behaviour common to all peoples, everywhere, throughout time, although the name and details may be culturally dependent, as will the value placed on the archetype. Compare the self-deprecatory answer 'Oh, I'm only a mother' given by many women these days to the question 'And what do you do?' with the honour and privilege accorded to a pregnant women in certain tribes, who are said to be carried everywhere and fed special food throughout her pregnancy.

The mother archetype involves the ability to bring forth new life and to nurture and care for the young. A person does not have to be a biological mother, or even a woman, for the mother archetype to be activated. The archetypes are potentials or collectively agreed frameworks for being a certain way in a certain situation. Many people who were neither young men nor particularly trained in combat or survival skills became heroes on the day of the London bombings. The situation activated the hero archetype. The wise person archetype comes in many guises – witch, wizard, shaman – all with the ability to move between worlds at will, to bless or curse and generally to do magic. This archetype is generally feared and ridiculed in our culture but may be re-emerging as an aspect of the healer archetype. The healer is the person who cures or fixes ailments. For several centuries now the Western healer has dealt mainly with the physical body, using an ever more sophisticated array of scientific and technological knowledge in support of his skill. The complementary therapy healer, particularly if she works with energy, may value her intuition as much as her rational logical understanding, may work to heal the emotional mental and energetic bodies as well, and may even utilise spirit guides, angels or channelled beings to help in her work.

Polarities

Many aspects of our experience contain a duality. Light and dark, night and day, up and down, black and white; one cannot exist without the other. If it were not for evil, we would have no concept of good. Every archetype also contains a polarity, two opposite and contrasting aspects. Consider man and woman, mother and child, angel and demon, persecutor and victim. The yin–yang symbol is a visual representation of this idea. Like the yin–yang symbol, we are all of us a mix of good and bad, saint and sinner, wisdom and foolishness. This is what makes us human beings, the fact that we are neither completely perfect nor entirely rotten. When one side of an archetype is activated in a situation, it requires the other polarity to be present too. When someone refuses to behave archetypically, things get confusing. There's a story about a priest who was held up at gunpoint one night in a dark alley. Without thinking, he held up a hand and said, 'Bless you, my son.' 'Thank you, father' said his attacker, and moved off. The priest didn't behave like a victim and not only broke that archetype; he introduced a new one into the situation and the other man switched from attacker to parishioner. (This was in America, where many more people are regular churchgoers.)

The doctor/patient archetype

Adolf Guggenbuhl-Craig, in his book about power in the helping professions (1971), describes the doctor/patient archetype, and why it might be important for those who work with the sick to examine how this archetype, which has attracted them to work in this area, might be operating in their own inner world. According to Jung (Jung 1993), the archetypal polarity exists internally as well. We all contain within us the potential to be priest and parishioner, for example, or parent and child, or doctor and patient. When one polarity is activated in the outer world, the other one is activated in the inner world, in the unconscious. The more a person identifies with one aspect of the archetype, the more she denies the possibility of the existence of the other within herself and the more likely she is to project this aspect onto others. We all find polarities hard to bear, and want certainty, but to split an archetype and say 'This is me, but this is certainly not me' gives a false reassurance.

Doctors and healers can project their inner sick person onto their clients, but so can our clients project their inner doctor or healer onto us, which can feel wonderful, since it enhances our power and status in their eyes, but can also be an unwelcome burden. There is a danger that the doctor/healer begins to believe that she is healthy and strong and the people she works with are sick and weak. Things that are repressed in the psyche have a tendency to gain energy. Someone shut in a cupboard will shout and hammer on the door until he is released, whereupon he may well have a word or two to say to whoever locked the door on him in the first place. In a similar way, material that is shut up in the unconscious because it is unacceptable or dangerous seeks to be let out and to destroy the good, acceptable stuff in the conscious part of the mind. This is what Jung called the shadow. The energy of the shadow in the doctor/healer archetype will try to destroy the good, positive, caring aspect. In order to stop this happening it is necessary for the doctor/healer to acknowledge the shadow, and their own inner patient/sick person.

✍ **Exercise to explore your healer/patient archetype**
The following exercise suggests a way to explore with these concepts for yourself. But first we need to talk about terminology. For doctor we could substitute therapist, healer, shaman, practitioner or our own professional label such as chiropractor, aromatherapist, or Rolfer. There are fewer

alternatives for patient, and with its connotations of passivity, many CAM therapists prefer the term client, implying as it does the contractual nature of the relationship, with the client having the financial power to choose her practitioner. There's an aspect of the term patient that, I think, has become devalued. Being unwell requires patience. The process of healing can't be rushed. Severe illness also requires a suspension of everyday life and entry into another world, where the patient surrenders to the business of being ill. Some CAM practitioners do use the word patient. Osteopaths treat patients rather than clients, and maybe this tradition derives from the medical origins of osteopathy. Invalid, customer, user, sufferer — these words are potential alternatives to patient or client. I will use the words healer and patient, but I'd like you to choose the words that fit best for you in this context.

Sit comfortably in a quiet room, with writing materials ready. Do whatever you usually do to settle into your body and still your mind.

Now imagine you are alone in a small film studio, facing a blank white screen. As you watch, some words appear on the screen. You read 'Your inner healer'. The words fade, to be replaced with an image. Take your time, don't censor, and see what emerges. Notice your reactions to the image. The screen goes blank and another title appears. It reads 'Your inner patient'. The words fade. Wait for an image to appear, trusting that whatever comes up is meant to be there. Notice your reactions. Let the image fade.

Come back slowly to the room and write about or draw the images and how you felt about each one. Work fast, allowing your thoughts to flow without censoring them. When you've finished, put it all to one side. Some time later, come back to the images and your reactions, and think about the implications for yourself as a practitioner. It may help to discuss the exercise with your supervisor or a colleague.

Here's what happened when I did the exercise.

My inner healer is a being of light, possibly with wings, but no body to speak of, just a light presence with a head, beard and long hair, a bit like Jesus Christ. But he's a contemporary Jesus who's waiting to appear on breakfast television. He's done this many times before. My inner patient is a disgusting heap of large intestine. Immediately I want to disown it and find a more comfortable image. But in my fantasy there it was as well, the pile of intestines, sitting on the other chair in the TV studio, waiting for the presenter's questions.

When I look for the meaning in the images, the split between them is obvious. My inner healer is good, pure and spiritual and my inner patient is disgusting, and not even fully human. I accept that I'd better do some work on my archetypes or I'm going to be in trouble!

Endings

The therapeutic relationship begins with a contract, an agreement about what will happen, what won't happen, where, when and how the agreed goals are to be reached. Ideally, when the relationship ends, when the treatment is over, the boundary needs to be sealed again, the ending acknowledged. Actors, or participants in a drama workshop, go through a process called de-roling, to remind themselves who they are, after playing a certain character: 'I am not a werewolf. I am Jimmy Smith.' 'I am not Lady Windermere. I am Sahida Kahn.' In an ideal world, practitioner and client can now, at the end of treatment, be Alan and Sara again. Or can they? Many psychotherapists would argue that the therapeutic relationship never ends, that the client always carries an imago of whoever the practitioner was for her, no matter what subsequent contact they may have. The power imbalance in the relationship doesn't end when the relationship ends; the practitioner always knows more about the client than the other way round and may have seen the client naked, or emotionally vulnerable.

Very little has been written about this subject in relation to CAM relationships, compared to the psychotherapy relationship where the ending is taken very seriously. This makes sense if you remember that therapist and client may have known each other over many years and a close attachment may have developed. But some of the reasons for paying attention still hold for a shorter and less intense CAM relationship. The ending is a time for unfinished business, a time to say the things that you might regret leaving unsaid, a time for appreciations and constructive feedback. For a CAM practitioner, the final session offers a chance to revisit the goals of the initial contract and discuss with the client if he feels they've been achieved, what helped and what didn't, and to talk about what he might do next. The ending is a time for expressions of loss or sadness, or gratitude, or other feelings that might arise. Psychotherapists acknowledge that an ending can trigger memories of other losses in a person's life. I'm not saying that after six acupuncture sessions a client will find herself in a state of mourning akin to when her mother died, but that it is something to bear in mind, for us as well as our clients. Our society finds death difficult, and we prefer to pass swiftly over moments of loss that remind us of the impermanence of all things. And yet, as practitioners, we are continually saying goodbye to people who have let us touch their lives. How do we do this without being touched ourselves? How do we harden our hearts to the constant losses?

The average number of sessions for a complementary therapy client to see a therapist is five or six, but there are some clients, and some therapies, where the relationship lasts much longer and an attachment develops. In these situations it is also worth remembering that the client may possibly experience the break in continuity of treatment that happens whenever one party has a holiday negatively. In my experience, many clients claim not to be at all bothered by the break and maybe that's true. Others may simply say, 'I missed you', and I know they felt the gap. Others communicate difficulty indirectly. Harry, for example, cancels his first session after the holidays and rearranges the second one. When we meet, I feel as if I can't get anything right. Everything I say is somehow wrong for him. I suspect he's cross with me for going away. And when Carol tells me about her summer adventures trekking in Greece I feel dead and bored and there's no connection between us. Although she's talking about exciting things I wonder if she's also communicating her loss of me in the holidays. With long-term clients, watch out for unusual behaviour around holiday breaks that may indicate that something is wrong and, if you think it would help, mention it lightly in conversation with your client. And then there's the biggest ending of them all…

Arrangements in the event of your death or an event that renders you incapable of working

Have you ever thought about what would happen to your clients if you had a sudden heart attack and died? Or if you were involved in a car accident, seriously injured with no prognosis as to when, if ever, you'd recover? People who die without a will often leave a big mess for their families to sort out. Reluctant as we are to think about such things, it does make good sense to put procedures in place to take care of your clients should the worst happen to you. Death and incapacity are two very different things. If you die, that's it, you're never going to work again – and your clients are never going to see you again. It's not possible to predict a client's reaction to a therapist's death, but there will be some emotional reaction, and, if the relationship is a close or longstanding one, the client may experience it as a personal bereavement. Often we don't know how much we matter to the people we work with. I remember being a bit shocked when someone told me, years after we'd finished working together, 'When I first came to London, you were my only friend. My week revolved around my appointment with you'.

SOME QUESTIONS TO CONSIDER WHEN PLANNING FOR YOUR DEATH

1. Who do you want to be your professional executor? That is, the person who takes responsibility for contacting, as soon as possible, your current clients to tell them the news. If you work in the NHS or in a clinic or health centre, an administrator or centre manager

may automatically take this responsibility. But if you work in private practice, you may want to have an arrangement, perhaps reciprocal, with a colleague. If you have a locum who covers your practice while you are on holiday, it makes sense to ask that person, because he or she will be known to some of your clients.

2. What information do you want to be offered to your clients? Details of a bereavement counselling service? Another practitioner who could see them in your place? Do you want them told about funeral arrangements? (Think of your family.)

3. What will happen to your client records in the event of your death?

4. If you work with client groups who are emotionally fragile and could be greatly disturbed by the news, is there someone who could offer immediate support?

INCAPACITY OF UNKNOWN DURATION

1. Who do you want to tell your clients? Remember, a family member may not be the best person if the situation is serious. Is this person willing to remain in communication with clients to inform them of changes in the situation?

2. What do you want them to know? Think hard about this – you may feel comfortable about the people you work with knowing you've been in a car accident, but not that you've been admitted to psychiatric hospital. You may feel it's appropriate for clients to have personal information or you may not.

3. Is there someone who could act as a locum until you recover and can work again?

CLIENT CONTACT DETAILS

The person chosen as your professional executor must have an up-to-date list of the people on your books, so that she can contact them as soon as possible to inform them. I know of one person who turned up for her counselling appointment at a clinic and was knocking on the door for about five minutes, before it was answered and she was told 'Oh didn't you know? X died two weeks ago'. The lack of sensitivity and inadequate communication left the person in question not only shocked and upset but angry. Would you want that to happen to your clients?

Closing thoughts

When someone asks what I do and I reply that I'm a psychotherapist, a not-uncommon and only half-joking response is to ask if I'm psychoanalysing the speaker, right there and then. This sort of reaction points to the notion that psychotherapists have some special and magical understanding to see into people's minds and read their thoughts. The aim of this chapter was to demystify psychotherapeutic thinking and to explain some key concepts very simply (too simply, some might say) and put them in a context that is relevant to the complementary therapist.

9
Working with Vulnerable Clients

Sarah was lying on the couch as usual and I was holding her skull, tuning into her fluid tides, noticing her breathing slow and her muscles soften when suddenly she was in startle response, muscles tensed and frozen, breathing stopped, eyes wide and staring. I felt a sudden resonating rush of adrenaline. 'What's happening, Sarah?' I asked. 'There's a huge knife, hanging over me. It's about to come down, right into me.' I recognised a trauma response, possibly relating to one of her periods of electroconvulsive shock treatment in her teenage years, but the main job at that moment wasn't to understand but to help her come back to the present and reduce her autonomic system arousal. 'Sarah, it's OK, it's not happening now, you're here with me. Can you hear my voice? Can you feel my hand on your shoulder? Yes, good. Now take a deep breath, that's good and another, let it all go. You're starting to shake, don't worry, it's OK, I'll get you a blanket…' and so on, in a calm monologue about her experience in the present, with the emphasis on somatic sensation, bringing her back from whatever it was that had frightened her so much.

All the variables pertaining to the therapeutic relationship need particular attention when we work with people from certain client groups; those with communication difficulties, learning disability, users of mental health services, people with physical disabilities, those who are terminally ill, victims of violence, people who are using or in recovery from drug or alcohol abuse, those in prison. Many people in these groups may also be suffering some degree of post-traumatic stress. Practitioners who choose to work with a particular client group would do well to read and research, take specialist training courses and find a supervisor with experience in the field.

Trust and safety can be issues, so boundary maintenance is important. A room where you and your client won't be disturbed, clarity of agreement about time, money, what will and won't happen in the treatment room may need to be reiterated more than once. Never assume that the other person's perception of the world is the same as yours. While this is true for all clients, it is especially so for those from vulnerable groups. Allow plenty of time for the client to talk, listen well and ask if you don't understand.

The power imbalance may be heightened, a vulnerable person being more dependent on the one who is less so. For example, someone with a hearing impairment has needs that a hearing person doesn't, for good light so he can see faces, for reduced surface noise and for the speaker to be clear and direct. As well as the reduction in power that comes with having special needs, people from vulnerable groups often have less power to make choices about their lives. If you've spent any time in hospital, you'll have had a taste of this. Your routine is dictated by hospital schedules, medical personnel decide when you stay in bed, when you can get up and go home and you may not even have choice about what you eat. People who have had a lifetime of being told what to do find it hard to know what they want, let alone communicate it. They may also have difficulty saying no to something they don't like.

The touch history of people who have had extensive institutionalised or medical touch can foster an expectation that physical contact is something to be endured, or that it may be painful, but rarely enjoyed. The ability to choose whether to be touched or not, what sort of touch and where may be lost. People who've received physical or sexual violence may have distorted perception of touch and find it hard to distinguish good and bad or sexual and non-sexual touch.

Unconscious process is likely to be activated, particularly splitting and projection. If we can't face and accept our deepest fears about disability, dependence, madness, ageing and death, if we leave our terrors untouched in our shadow, the burden of holding our split-off and unacknowledged beliefs and feelings becomes, yet again, the burden of the person in the wheelchair, the woman at death's door, the man living with schizophrenia.

Guidelines for working with people who are physically vulnerable

The umbrella term 'physically vulnerable' includes people with physical impairment (temporary, like a fractured femur in a plaster cast, or permanent, like a limb affected by polio) and/or disability (paralysis from birth injury or accident), and frailty arising from a debilitating illness (chronic fatigue syndrome), or from extreme age. If you have ever broken an arm or leg or put one hand out of action by cutting a finger, if you can remember the complete lethargy that follows a bout of flu, then you have a slight idea of what it is like to live with physical vulnerability – except that for most people who are physically vulnerable life is like that all the time. Imagine the frustration, shame or embarrassment of being slower, or less able than others, or what it must be like to depend on carers for help with dressing or feeding or walking. Imagine what it must feel like to look unusual, or be stared at, to feel different from others and afraid of being judged. Imagine how it feels living with a condition which you know will deteriorate and eventually be the cause of your death. We need to be sensitive to the emotional and psychological aspects of living with a physical impairment. On the one hand, we can't relate to the person as if he were able bodied, and on the other we can't assume that we know what it's like to live in his body. Just because he is slower or needs assistance, he is not a child – don't infantilise. It helps to be aware of your own reaction to and feelings about physical impairment.

People who have needed a lot of medical attention such as operations, periods in hospital, nursing care, or physiotherapy will have had considerable experience of being touched in a particular way. Without wanting to imply that all health-care professionals are lacking in sensitivity, there is a way that patients can be treated as if they were just bodies, and faulty bodies at that. There may be little choice about being touched, or refusing painful or uncomfortable touch. If you use physical contact it may be helpful to explain to the client that it is not meant to be uncomfortable and that he can make choices about how he is touched and where.

If you are working in a private practice or a salon or health centre, in other words any environment that is not specifically designed to cater for the needs of physically vulnerable people, then a rough assessment of need in relation to the facilities available should be made prior to the first attendance. It's no use to a wheelchair user to arrive for a session and find that the treatment room is on the fourth floor. If the client needs to undress, allow more time for this and for the initial consultation. Be prepared to adapt how you work and negotiate with your client about where would be most comfortable for the treatment – in a chair or on the couch – and how to position and support her body. Remember that if there is sensory loss she may not be able to give accurate feedback. If she has equipment with her, like a wheelchair, braces, breathing apparatus or even walking stick, ask where she would like them to be during the treatment. If she has incontinence problems, be sensitive to potential embarrassment, and straightforward about discussing practical possibilities.

Guidelines for working with people who have sensory impairment

Visual impairment

Practical issues to bear in mind when working with visually impaired clients are to keep the layout of the room the same if possible and inform the client if items have been changed around. Avoiding moving the client's possessions. Ask if he would prefer to remove contact lenses or glasses, and with the latter, if he would like them close by during the treatment. If someone cannot see what you are doing, or what you want him to do, talk it through clearly. Maybe talk about what you are doing during the treatment, especially on a first visit. Ask him how much assistance he would like moving around the room and getting on and off the couch.

Hearing impairment

Some hearing impaired people use British Sign Language to communicate, and some wear hearing aids, and most lip read. The speech of a hearing impaired person may be hard to follow if she was born deaf or became deaf before she learned to speak. At all times, make sure your face is visible so that the person can lip read easily. Keep your face in the light, don't cover your mouth with your hand and speak clearly. If the person has a 'good' ear, position yourself to speak to that side. Ask if your client wants to remove her aids during the treatment, and then remember that she won't be able to hear you at all. Negotiate prearranged signs for 'turn over now' or for your client to use to signal discomfort.

Guidelines for working with people with communication difficulty

Communication involves the ability to understand language and the ability to produce meaningful speech. A person with a learning difficulty may be affected in both areas, but a person who has lost the use of his muscles of speech production, which can happen after a stroke or for a person with multiple sclerosis or Parkinson's disease, may have perfect comprehension. Someone with dementia may have both abilities but her short-term memory loss means she can't remember what has just been said. The relational aspects of the whole treatment need special consideration for clients with communication difficulties. He may not be able to understand you, or you may not be able to understand him, or both. He may be accompanied by a family member, carer or advocate, to speak for him, in which case you need to be sensitive to issues of confidentiality, and to include the client as much as possible in the consultation, to avoid a 'Does he take sugar?' situation.

Ascertain if the client has difficulty with comprehension or speech. If the former, establish an appropriate method of communication. Face the client and make use of facial expression and gesture, and use simple language. This would be inappropriate and infantilising in a person with good understanding. If the problem is in speech production, allow time, ask for clarification and repeat what's been said to check if you've got it right. Don't pretend to understand if you don't, and use writing, if appropriate.

Explain as clearly as you can what will happen. If your client has a history of extensive medical treatment or currently lives in an institution, she may not be used to making choices about her treatment, so try to establish that you expect her to do this and be sensitive to what she seems to want. If she has a history of painful or invasive treatments, she may be anxious about any physical contact, so go slowly. It may help to establish a simple signal, like raising a hand, for the client to use for 'this is not OK', so that she has a simple way to let you know during the treatment if she's uncomfortable. Be sensitive to changes in autonomic nervous system responses, and other non-verbal cues, in the client while you are working. Allow more time for aftercare as well as for the initial consultation.

Post-traumatic stress

A traumatic event is one that is an actual or perceived threat to a person's life or sense of bodily integrity, or one that involves witnessing acts of violence to others. This might include rape, being taken hostage, being in a train crash, losing one's home in a natural disaster, or witnessing a murder. A traumatic event doesn't necessarily traumatise a person: many people have the resilience to deal with an awful thing happening, to process it and move on. When this can't happen, the individual is at risk of developing post-traumatic stress or post-traumatic stress disorder (PTSD). The difference is that the latter condition disrupts normal functioning.

The physiological reaction to any traumatic event that is overwhelming is very specific; both the fight and flight (sympathetic system) and the relaxation branches (parasympathetic system) of the autonomic nervous system are activated together, resulting in 'freezing', sometimes called tonic immobility. The feeling is of being like a rabbit caught in the headlights of a car, unable to move. Both emotional reactions and muscular reactions are frozen. In someone suffering from PTSD it is as if the feelings appropriate to the situation – terror, rage, hurt – never had a chance to be acknowledged, and have remained trapped in the body. Similarly, the appropriate behavioural response to the situation – to fight back, scream, run away – remain held, resulting in chronic muscular contractions in the relevant skeletal muscles.

PTSD is more common following childhood trauma. Children lack the resources to understand and deal with traumatic events. If the trauma is of human design, as in the case of childhood abuse, then the effects are much more long-lasting. A person abused as a child finds it difficult to distinguish good internal body sensations from bad ones, and may use disassociation, or cutting off from the body, as a way of coping. Hyperarousal of the autonomic nervous system is common, and symptoms of PTSD resulting from this include insomnia, anxiety states, digestive disturbance and difficulties in concentration.

There are a number of factors arising from childhood abuse or trauma, or from adult trauma, that affect how such a person receives or interprets touch. Because of the way the whole nervous system is 'conditioned' by trauma, any event in the present that reminds the person, consciously or not, can trigger the original physiological reaction. In extreme cases, it is as if the whole event is happening right here and now, in present time. This is called a flashback. In less extreme reactions, a trigger may elicit a state of anxiety and fear, for no apparent reason. If the original trauma involved touch, or bodily contact from the abuser, it follows that touch – even the innocent caring touch of a complementary therapist – can trigger a traumatic reaction in the body.

Another factor concerns body posture, or somatic memory. If the original trauma involved having to lie still, without making a sound – the conditions that many clients and practitioners assume as natural for receiving a treatment – then assuming that position in present time may act as a trigger. If the abusing person was also a loved parent, the person may have developed confusion about good and bad touch, may assume that painful touch is normal, or be unable to distinguish between, say, pleasant and painful pressure on the muscles. If the abuse was sexual, there may also be confusion between non-sexual and sexualised touch.

Finally, someone suffering from PTSD, for whatever reason, may find the whole experience of a therapeutic treatment involving physical contact so unsettling that she may resort to the survival strategy common to many traumatised people, which is to dissociate, leaving the body behind, and wandering off somewhere else – in an extreme form, this may involve literally leaving the body, and watching proceedings from above. More usually, it might mean taking refuge in the mind, thinking about other things, engaging the therapist in trivial chat. To a sensitive therapist, the body of someone in a disassociated state feels as if, literally, there is no one home.

Guidelines for working with people with PTSD

The work of Babette Rothschild (2000), an international trauma therapist, is essential reading for suggestions for working safely in this area. She points out that it helps to be very familiar with the physiology of the stress and trauma response, both as a means of recognising sympathetic nervous system arousal and to be able to teach fight, flight and freeze. Signs that the client is showing heightened arousal indicate that all is not well (this is true for any client, not just those with PTSD). Watch for changes in breathing and heart rate, skin colour, and sweating. Notice your own somatic responses; if you feel heightened muscle tension or anxiety with no apparent external cause, you may be resonating with your client's arousal. Aim to reduce arousal by taking the client away from whatever is going on in his inner world, thereby altering his autonomic nervous system response. The following suggestions might help:

- Remind him to breathe.

- Ask him to clench and release his hands.

- Ask him to look round the room and name what he sees.

- Change the subject to something with neutral content.

In the longer term, teach him about strawberries and resources (see Chapter 2) and how to use them to reduce hyperarousal. This is where the ability to teach the physiology of stress is helpful. People suffering PTSD, as well as those who have panic or anxiety attacks, often believe that there is something seriously wrong with them, or that they're going crazy, and are reassured by factual information that explains what is happening in their bodies, and that the symptoms they experience are actually normal responses.

Issues of trust and safety are very important and it helps the client if you are very clear about your boundaries, and maintain a professional relationship. Be clear about time and money as well. Negotiate with your client about the treatment and discuss options. Be explicit about what you will do and stick to it.

It may help to establish a prearranged signal for 'stop now' or 'that's enough' and practise it before you begin the treatment so your client can trust that you will use it. Consider using a running commentary as you work. 'I'm going to rest my hands here for a moment, and then I'll uncover your back and start to oil your skin.' Keep comments neutral. The client may want to keep her eyes open. Be flexible. The most important thing is her feeling of safety.

Survivors of sexual or physical abuse may have difficulty recognising the difference between sexual and non-sexual touch, or between nurturing and abusive touch. All the suggestions for working with someone with post-traumatic stress apply, and it can be helpful, if the client becomes anxious during the treatment, to actually state that you are not going to hit her, touch her inappropriately or hurt her. Be sensitive and use your discretion. Survivors may also have difficulties with the idea of lying down, or removing clothes. Be prepared to be flexible.

Chemical dependency

The whole subject of chemical dependency and abuse is loaded with questions and value judgements. At what point does alcohol use stop being social drinking and become alcoholism? Why is addiction to a legal substance like caffeine more acceptable than addiction to cocaine? When does use of a substance become abuse? Excessive consumption of any substance can be injurious to health and as complementary therapists we are concerned with the general well being of our clients, but we have to be careful not to assume a client has a substance problem if he hasn't indicated as much, and to be aware of our own feelings about the issue, and to walk a fine line between offering support and telling a client what we think he should do. This client group can test our ability to be empathetic and offer unconditional positive regard. It helps to remember that the behaviour and the person doing it are not the same. In that way it becomes possible to respect the person without condoning his drug or alcohol use.

If a client arrives for a session under the influence of alcohol or non-prescribed drugs, treatment is usually contraindicated, to protect the practitioner as well as the client.

What to do if a client starts crying

Emotional release can be a normal outcome from many kinds of therapeutic treatments. Joyce Vetterlein, an osteopath with many years' experience, says that nowadays the public perception of her therapy and how it works is pretty accurate – with one exception. Many clients are surprised when there is an emotional element, when they find themselves in tears or wanting to hit somebody. They don't see the connection between the mind and the body. But, as Joyce tells them, 'the body remembers everything' (Private conversation 2005).

If you notice tears leaking or trickling out of the eyes with little noticeable change in breathing, ask 'you OK?' or 'like a tissue?'. Let your client know that you've noticed but keep your response light and neutral. You don't have to stop. If your client begins to sob or cry noisily during the treatment, tell her you're going to stop for a while, and ask her to curl on her side. This is easier for breathing and usually feels safer. Offer tissues. If it happens during the consultation, again offer tissues and sit and wait. You might want to put a hand on her arm or hand until she quietens, but first ask whether the touch is to comfort the client or yourself. You don't have to do anything. She may want to talk about it and, if so, all you have to do is listen. You don't have to make it all right – that isn't your job.

When the tears have subsided ask her what she'd like and whether to continue with the treatment. Offer water. Ascertain, if you don't already know, whether she has professional help or someone to talk to. If appropriate, offer a referral to a counselling or psychotherapy agency.

Note

Some of the material in this chapter has already appeared in *Practical Pathology for the Massage Therapist* by Su Fox (2004).

Summary

At the start of this book we met a woman who, in one scenario, was so caught up in her preoccupations that she was oblivious to her surroundings. In the next she appears grounded, present and mindful of her environment and able to name and appreciate the flowers around her. In the last, it's as if she's moved beyond the duality of existence into an experience of total connectedness.

Like the woman, we've learned, on our journey through this book, that it pays to give attention to the therapeutic relationship, because it plays a crucial part of the healing process. Like the woman, we've grounded and centred, learned to be mindful and to focus, thought about the core conditions for forming a good alliance. We considered the importance of listening and communication skills. We understood why boundaries matter so much. And then, like her, we moved beyond the realm of factual materiality to explore notions of power and sexuality. We thought about the impact of touch, and about unconscious process and how this may need attention in the therapeutic relationship.

And, in the end, we arrive back at the beginning, where we started; practitioner and client together in the treatment room, one of them a little wiser in the ways of the therapeutic relationship.

References

The Accupuncture Council's Code of Professional Conduct. Accessed on 8 October 2007 at: www.acupuncture.org.uk/content/resources/codeofprofessionalconduct.pdf.

Balens, D. (2004) 'When Your Client Can't Get No Satisfaction.' *Shiatsu Society News.* Winter.

Bloom, W. (2001) *The Endorphin Effect.* London: Piatkus.

British Medical Association (2004) *Medical Ethics Today.* London: BMJ Books.

Clarkson, P. (1995) *The Therapeutic Relationship: In Psychoanalysis, Counselling, Psychology and Psychotherapy.* London: Whurr.

Code of Ethics (2004) The Craniosacral Therapy Association of the UK. London: Craniosacral Therapy Association. Available at www.craniosacral.co.uk/files/ethics.pdf.

Collins English Dictionary (1998) Glasgow: HarperCollins.

Damasio, A. (2000) *The Feeling of What Happens: Body, Emotion and the Making of Consciousness.* London: Vintage.

Dunn, D. (2000) 'The Year's Afternoon.' In *The Year's Afternoon.* London: Faber and Faber.

Fox, S. (2004) *Practical Pathology for the Massage Therapist.* Lydney: Corpus Publishing.

Gendlin, E.T. (1978) *Focusing.* Toronto: Bantam.

Gibran, K. (2002) *The Prophet.* London: Penguin.

Guggenbuhl-Craig, A. (1971) *Power in the Helping Professions.* New York, NY: Spring Publications.

Hubble, M.M., Duncan, B.L. and Miller, S.D. (1999) *Heart and Soul of Change: What Works in Therapy.* Washington, DC: American Psychological Association.

Hunter, M. and Struve, J. (1998) *The Ethical Use of Touch in Psychotherapy.* Thousand Oaks, CA: Sage.

Jehu, D. (1994) *Patients as Victims: Sexual Abuse in Psychotherapy and Counselling.* Chichester: John Wiley.

Jung, C.G. (1993) *Memories, dreams, reflections.* London: Fontana Press.

Kelner, M.J. (2000) 'The therapeutic relationship under fire.' In M. Kelner, B. Wellman, B. Pescosolido and M. Saks (eds) *Complementary and Alternative Medicine: Challenge and Change.* Amsterdam: Gordon and Breach.

Layard, Lord. (2006) 'The Depression Report: A New Deal for Depression and Anxiety Disorders.' Paper presented at The London School of Economics and Political Science, London, June 2006. Accessed on 8 October 2007 at: http://cep.lse.ac.uk/research/mentalhealth.

Lee-Treweek, G., Heller, T., Katz, J., Stone, J. and Spurr, S. *Perspectives on Complementary and Alternative Medicine.* London: Routledge.

Macbeth, J. (2002) *Moon over Water. Meditation Made Clear with Techniques for Beginners and Initiates.* Bath: Gateway.

Mann, D. (1997) *Psychotherapy: An Erotic Relationship.* London: Routledge.

The Massage Training Institute Code of Ethics (2007). Available online at www.massagetraining.co.uk/ethics.php.

Mitchell, A. and Cormack, M. (1998) *The Therapeutic Relationship in Complementary Health Care.* Edinburgh: Churchill Livingstone.

Myss, C. (2004) 'The Call to Live a Symbolic Life'. A live workshop on four CDs. Carlsback, CA: Hay House.

Nhat Hanh, T. (1998) *Teachings on Love.* Berkeley, CA: Parallex Press.

Niebuhr, R. (1986) *The Essential Reinhold Niebuhr: Selected Essays and Addresses.* London: Yale University Press.

Oleson, A.K. (2004) *In Your Hands* (Forbrydelser). Denmark: Ib Tardini.

Orbach, S. (1999) *The Impossibility of Sex.* London: Allen Lane.

Rogers, C.R. (1951) Client-centred Therapy. Boston, MA: Houghton Mifflin.

Rosenberg, J.L. with Rand, M.L. and Asay, D. (1985) *Body, self and soul.* Atlanta, GA: Humanics.

Rosenberg, M.B. (2005) 'Nonviolent Communication: A Language of Compassion.' Speech given at The Breath of Life Conference organised by The Craniosacral Therapy Association, on 25 May 2005 at the Brunei Gallery, London.

Rothschild, B. (2000) *The Body Remembers.* New York, NY: W.W. Norton.

Rothschild, B. and Rand, M. (2006) Help for the helper: The psychophysiology of compasion fatigue and vicarious trauma. New York, NY: W.W. Norton.

Ryan, J. (ed.) (2005) *How Does Psychotherapy Work?* London: Karnac.

Sheldrake, R. (2003) *The Sense of Being Stared At.* London: Crown Publishing Group.

Smith, E.W.L., Clance, P.R. and Imes, S. (eds) (1998) *Touch in Psychotherapy: Theory, Research and Practice.* New York, NY: Guilford Press.

Stone, J. and Katz, J. (2005) 'The therapeutic relationship and complementary and alternative medicine.' In T. Heller (ed.) *Perspectives on Complementary and Alternative Medicine.* London: Routledge.

Vetterlein, J. (2004) Comments made in private conversation.

Wall, P. (1999) *Pain: The Science of Suffering.* London: Weidenfeld and Nicolson.

Recommended Reading

Balens, D. (Winter 2004) 'When your client can't get no satisfaction.' Shiatsu Society News. Rugby: The Shiatsu Society.

Benjamin, A. (1981, 3rd edn) *The Helping Interview*. Boston: Houghton Mifflin Co.

Bloom, W. (2001) *The Endorphin Effect: A breakthrough strategy for holistic health and spiritual wellbeing*. London: Piatkus Books Ltd.

British Medical Association. (2002, 2nd edn) *Medical Ethics Today: The BMA's Handbook of Ethics and Law*. London: BMJ Publishing Group.

Clarkson, Petruska. (1995) *The Therapeutic Relationship: In Psychoanalysis, Counselling Psychology and Psychotherapy*. San Diego, CA: Singular Publishing Group.

Collins English Dictionary: Millennium Edition (1998, 4th edn). London: HarperCollins.

Damasio, A. (2000) *The Feeling of What Happens: Body, Emotion and the Making of Consciousness*. London: Vintage.

Dunn, D. (2000) 'The Year's Afternoon.' In *The Year's Afternoon*. London: Faber and Faber.

Fox, S. (2004) *Practical Pathology for the Massage Therapist*. Lydney: Corpus Publishing Ltd.

Gendlin, E. T. (1978) *Focusing*. New York, NY: Bantam Dell Publishing.

Gibran, K. (2002) *The Prophet*. London: Penguin.

Graham, H. (1998) *Complementary Therapies in Context: The Psychology of Healing*. London: Jessica Kingsley Publishers.

Guggenbuhl-Craig, A. (1971) *Power in the Helping Professions*. New York, NY: Spring Publications.

Hubble, M. M., Duncan, B. L. and Miller, S. D. (eds) (1999) *The Heart and Soul of Change: What Works in Therapy*. Washington, DC: American Psychological Association.

Hunter, M. and Struve, J. (1997) *The Ethical Use of Touch in Pschotherapy*. London: Sage Publications.

Jehu, D. (ed.) (1994) *Patients as Victims: Sexual Abuse in Psychotherapy and Counselling*. London: John Wiley.

Kelner, M.J. (2000) 'The Therapeutic Relationship Under Fire.' In M. Kelner, B. Wellman, B. Pescosolido and M Saks (eds) *Complementary and Alternative Medicine: Challenge and Change*. Amsterdam: Harwood Academic Publishers / Gordon and Breach.

Lee-Treweek, G., Heller, T., Katz, J., Stone, J. and Spurr, S. (eds) (2005) *Perspectives on Contemporary and Alternative Medicine*. New York, NY: Routledge/Open University Press.

Macbeth, J. (2002) *Moon Over Water: Meditation Made Clear with Techniques for Beginners and Initiates.* Bath: Gateway Books.

Mann, D. (1997) *Psychotherapy – An Erotic Relationship: Transference and Countertransference Passions.* New York, NY: Routledge.

Mitchell, A. and Cormack, M. (1998) *The Therapeutic Relationship in Complementary Health Care.* London: Churchill Livingstone.

Myss, C. (2004) The Call to Live a Symbolic Life: A Live Workshop! (Audio CD). London: Hay House.

Nhat Hanh, T. (1998) *Teachings on Love.* Berkeley, CA: Parallax Press.

Orbach, S. (2002) *The Impossibility of Sex.* New York, NY: Touchstone/Simon & Schuster.

POPAN (2005) Clients' experience of Boundary Violations. Workshop at UKCP Ethics Day Conference.

Rogers, C. (2003) *On Becoming a Person: A Therapist's View of Psychotherapy.* London: Constable and Robinson.

Rosenberg, J. L., Rand, M. L. and Asay, D. (1985) *Body, Self and Soul.* Lake Worth, FL: Humanics Publishing Group.

Rothschild, B. (2000) *The Body Remembers: The Psychophysiology of Trauma and Trauma Treatment.* New York, NY: W.W. Norton & Co.

Ryan, J. (ed.) (2005) *How Does Psychotherapy Work?* London: Karnac Books.

Scott, T. (2003) *Integrative Psychotherapy in Healthcare: A Humanistic Approach.* New York, NY: Palgrave Macmillan.

Sheldrake, R. (2004) *The Sense of Being Stared.* New York, NY: Three Rivers Press / The Crown Publishing Group.

Smith, D. L. (1999) *Approaching Psychoanalysis: An Introductory Course.* London: Karnac Books.

Smith, E. W. L., Clance, P. R. and Imes, S. (eds) (1998) *Touch in Psychotherapy: Theory, Research and Practice.* New York, NY: Guilford Press.

Staunton, T. (ed) (2002) *Body Psychotherapy: Advancing Theory in Therapy.* New York, NY: Brunner-Routledge.

Stone, J. and Katz, J. (2005) 'The therapeutic relationship and complementary and alternative medicine.' In T. Heller (ed.) *Perspectives on Complementary and Alternative Medicine.* London: Routledge.

Turp, M. (2001) *Psychosomatic Health: The Body and the Word.* New York, NY: Palgrave Macmillan.

Wall, P. (1999) *Pain: The Science of Suffering.* London: Weidenfeld & Nicolson.

White, K. (ed.) (2004) *Touch, Attachment and the Body.* London: Karnac Books.

Subject Index

Note: The letter 'f' after a page
number denotes a figure

abused people 162, 163, 164–5
   see also sexual abuse; traumatised
      people; violent touch
acceptance 95, 96–8
accidental touch 121
Acupuncture Council 70
aerobic exercise 34, 35
aggression *see* aggressive touch;
      physically abused people;
      sexual abuse; traumatised
      people
aggressive touch 118
air 34, 35
alcoholism 165
anchors 39
anxiety 101
archetypal shadow 145
archetypes 150–3
assertiveness, in client communication
      94–5
attention 83–4, 85
authenticity 94, 95, 99
autonomic nervous system 64–5,
      162, 163, 164
awareness 15
   see also self awareness; somatic
      awareness

babies 143–4
'being real' 96, 99
   see also authenticity; real
      relationships
bereavement 155, 156
biology and sex 126–7
blind and visually impaired people
      161
body
   self care 34–40
   as therapeutic tool 46–7
   thoughts and feelings, responses
      to 138–9
   see also autonomic nervous system;
      centering; emotional
      responses; feelings;

focusing; grounding; mind;
      mindfulness; personal space;
      posture; psyche; somatic
      awareness; somatic
      countertransference; somatic
      memory
boundaries
   client contracts 16, 59–62, 80,
      81
   concept of 56–7
   confidentiality 62, 72, 80, 81–2,
      162
   crossing, by CAM practitioners
      72–3, 74–5
   disclosure 76–9
   importance 19
   laws 60–1, 79–81, 82
   malpractice and negligence 73,
      80–1, 82
   overlapping (dual relationships)
      68–72
   personal 63–8, 121–3
   physical 57–9
   record keeping and records 80,
      81–2, 156
   violation, by CAM practitioners
      72, 73–4, 121
   violation, by clients 75–6, 123
   vulnerable client groups 158–9,
      164
British Association of Counselling
      and Psychotherapy (BACP) 45
British Medical Association (BMA)
      70
Buddhism 11, 12, 94, 98, 113
burn out 46

CAM practitioners
   bad client experiences with 10,
      17–18, 30–1
   and bad clients 31, 32
   communication skills (*see*
      communication skills)
   endings 154–6
   good client experiences with 31
   and good clients 31
   personal boundaries 63–7

projections about 148–9
projections by 147–8
self awareness (*see* self awareness)
sexual contact with former clients
      131, 132–3, 134
carers 161–2
centering 48–9, 114
chemical dependency 165
childhood trauma 163
Christianity 113
cleanliness 58, 59, 80
cleansing rituals 59
client contracts 16, 59–62, 80, 81
clients
   bad clients 31–2
   bad experiences with CAM
      practitioners 10, 17–18,
      30–1
   bad experiences with healthcare
      professionals 29–31
   boundaries, violation by 75–6,
      123
   boundaries of 67–8, 72–5
   communication, assertiveness of
      94–5
   complaints by 73–4, 79–81
   contact details 156
   contracts 16, 59–62, 80, 81
   difficulties with 105–8
   endings 154–6
   former clients, sexual contact with
      practitioners 131–4
   good clients 31
   good experiences with CAM
      practitioners 31
   good experiences with healthcare
      professionals 31
   projections 148–50
   questioning by 66–7
   transference 25–6, 133–4,
      139–40
   see also distressed clients;
      vulnerable client groups
codes of conduct, professional 40,
      70, 79, 125
codes of ethics, professional 79, 125

172

Author Index